Testimonials

In 1968, a promising young physician, newly married and just beginning his medical career, is stricken with a mysterious neurologic illness for which he is hospitalized for months. He and his family live in fear that he will never be able to practice medicine again or provide for his family.

The Flashing Light: A Medical Mystery Memoir is the harrowing and ultimately inspiring story of Dr. Irving Fox's ordeal and dramatic recovery. It is also the story of his search for answers, 50 years later, to finally understand what had happened, and how he had overcome fear and uncertainty to become a highly regarded academic physician and successful pharmaceutical executive. Dr. Fox's compelling story is a testament to resiliency and hope, a light for others who may also be facing terrifying life events.

Catherine Milch MD
Vice-president, Immunology R&D
CSL Behring (King of Prussia, PA)

The Flashing Light: A Medical Mystery Memoir keeps you glued to the page trying to figure out what exactly was causing Irving Fox's terrifying symptoms at the young age of 25. This medical "whodunit" brings you inside Irving's inner turmoil and the medical mystery (with simplified explanations of medical jargon) as his doctors catapulted from one diagnosis to another.

Knowing Irving from my work in the Takeda Leadership Academy I could never have guessed that his past contained such a traumatic moment. It is lucky for all of us that he came through the experience and brought his wisdom to help others escape their own diagnostic nightmares.

Deborah Ancona,
Seley Distinguished Professor of Management,
MIT Sloan School of Management, and Founder
of the MIT Leadership Center.

When we think about the people we meet along our professional pathways, we should recognize with humility that we only know a fraction of the story of their journey to a crossroads with us.

In *The Flashing Light: A Medical Mystery Memoir*, Dr. Irving Fox reveals a series of events that could have completely changed the course of his future path to becoming the physician, professor, drug developer, mentor, and esteemed colleague that he has been to so many people, fortunately including me.

Our winding roads merged at Millennium/Takeda Pharmaceuticals (2005-2020) where we built a strong partnership based on mutual respect as colleagues, empathy for patients, and shared accountability for success as leaders. But, never could I have imagined anything like the story of *The Flashing Light* as a part of what filled Irving's deep reservoir of resilience, perseverance, and commitment to the advancement of medicine.

Karen Wolf, LLC
Consulting Practice focused on
BioPharma Team and Leadership Excellence

In *The Flashing Light: A Medical Mystery Memoir*, Irving Fox explores the mysterious neurological illness that fifty years earlier nearly derailed what would be a brilliant medical career. Building on his years as a teacher of medicine, Fox patiently and clearly explains the tests and treatments he underwent, providing a compelling first-person perspective on both the human and technical aspects of the patient experience. All was accomplished through painstaking reconstruction using his contemporaneous personal journal, hospital records, and interviews with those who witnessed this devastating period in his life. What emerges is an insightful look at what it means to suffer a severe illness for which specific treatments are not available. Most importantly, this book carries the lesson of the importance of hope in the face of even the greatest personal challenges.

David Eidelman,
Vice Principal and Dean, Faculty of Medicine
and Health Sciences, McGill University

I was a patient of Dr. Irving Fox beginning in January of 1981 until he resigned from the University of Michigan Medical Center. I had no idea he had gone through medical and emotional struggles of his own until recently, upon reading the content of his book, *The Flashing Light: A Medical Mystery Memoir*. However, reading his book about his health struggles explained for me a lot of his professional attributes and what helped make him the doctor and human being that he became. He has always been kind, thoughtful, caring, and compassionate. He always wanted the very best for me, not just medically speaking, but as a whole complete person. He treated other patients at the University of Michigan with the same wonderful qualities as he treated me in my experiences with him.

Mary Grimmette
Patient

Dr. Irving Fox is modest, self-disciplined, and hard-working, and has been gifted with a brilliant medical mind. I know this because for more than 60 years he has been my loyal and trusted friend. It was evident from an early age that he was destined for great accomplishments. Dr. Fox not only graduated first in his class from McGill University's medical school but also won many honours and distinctions. A 25-year-old Dr. Fox was struck by an unknown neurological illness that almost ended his career. Those of us who knew and loved him were devastated. In his book *The Flashing Light: A Medical Mystery Memoir*, Dr. Fox takes us through his remarkable recovery. Dr. Fox recovered totally and was able to embark on a very distinguished career, developing new drugs that improved the lives of thousands of patients. He authored and co-authored over 130 medical articles and contributed to more than 50 chapters in medical textbooks. Reading *The Flashing Light: A Medical Mystery Memoir* should provide help, guidance, and hope to those who need it.

Dr. Leonard Diamond,
DDS, DIP Perio, practitioner and lecturer
in Periodontics and Dental Implants

Author and Doctor Irving Fox takes us on his personal journey beginning in 2020 to chronicle through memory and existing medical records his own personal and mysterious health setback at the very beginning of his career in 1968 when he was a resident at Royal Victoria Hospital in Montreal. Fox intersperses his saga with simple-to-understand explanations of complex medical terms, brain processes, and pathologies, with humor and humility.

We marvel at Fox's ability to describe his relentless, if time-defined, pain and suffering as merely "unpleasant" and "uncomfortable"—a reflection of his resilient spirit. He offers his perspective on the artistry and also the limitations of even the most proficient medical providers, who integrate their knowledge and experience to find the source of symptoms and a correct diagnosis, "like piecing together a multi-dimensional jigsaw puzzle, working without a picture of the result." We sense that this author moved through his traumatic health episode and his life journey guided by the WWII British poster motto highlighted in chapter 6: "Keep calm and carry on"—a lesson in hope for our times.

Rabbi Jan Katz
Temple B'nai Israel, Laconia, New Hampshire

The Flashing Light: A Medical Mystery Memoir is a riveting, true-life story of the strange and mysterious illness that befell the author Irving Fox during his medical residency in the 1960s. Dr. Fox tells the story of his journey, now 50 years later, with insight from his medical training and his life experiences.

The onset of mysterious neurological and psychiatric symptoms early in his career and marriage had the potential to significantly upend his trajectory in life. Since that time, Irving has led a successful and distinguished career in academic medicine and in drug development, impacting thousands of patients' lives through his work in developing drugs for neurologic and inflammatory conditions. I have had the pleasure of working with Dr. Fox, who mentored me in my career. Reading this book gave me insights into the impact that this early experience had on shaping his life and his commitment to helping patients and developing young people in their careers.

Nancy Simonian, MD, CEO of Syros Pharmaceuticals

Reading Irving Fox's memoir of a haunting episode from his young adulthood brings to light the stark contrast between the advances of neuroscience of the past half-century, and the enigmas that continue to persist, particularly insofar as concerns the human mind. I devoured the chapters of *The Flashing Light: A Medical Mystery Memoir* with great enthusiasm, as they provide a glimpse of a younger man, with his entire future in front of him. Coming to know him later in life, I can still appreciate the influence this health struggle had on how he thinks and carries himself to this day. In his memoir, Fox freely shares important life lessons including the sudden departure of logic that accompanies the physician becoming the patient, as well as the relative inability to think rationally in matters that concern one's own health.

These imparted tidbits of wisdom carry a greater meaning when one imagines oneself in Fox's shoes, institutionalized in that era, at the mercy of an unexplained illness without a definitive diagnosis or obvious therapy. Fox is a scholar, a gentleman, a scientist, a physician, a drug developer, a mentor, and, most importantly, a friend. His lasting contributions to the professional growth and career development of others, myself included, have not gone unnoticed in the Boston biopharma world. It was a privilege to read this biographical narrative.

Asit Parikh MD PhD
CEO of MOMA Therapeutics

I am delighted to write in support of Dr Irving Fox and his new book, The Flashing Light: A Medical Mystery Memoir. I first met and began to work with Irving on July 1, 1969 when he arrived at Duke University to participate as a fellow in training in the Research Training Program. Most of his time over the next 2 years would be to do basic biomedical research in my laboratory in the Department of Medicine. I was unaware of his devastating and mysterious illness from which he had just recovered when we first met and I only learned of it recently, some 50 years later.

From the time we first met, I was very impressed with his superb medical training, and his intellectual skills. From the very outset, he was a quick learner and able to apply these newly acquired skills to the design of complex experimental approaches to solve problems and to reach appropriate conclusions. Not only was I very impressed at the beginning of our scientific relationship, but this matured over the next twenty years as we both moved up the academic ladder. On completion of his training in my lab, I strongly recommended him for a faculty position in the Department of Medicine at the University of Toronto, which he accepted in the early 1970s.

In 1975, I accepted the position as Chairman of the Department of Internal Medicine at the University of Michigan. One of my first recruitments was to bring Irving and his family to Ann Arbor for him to run the NIH-sponsored Clinical Research Center. He came in July, 1976, as its Associate Director and moved up in the summer of 1977 to become the Director. He held this position until he departed for a major leadership position in the pharmaceutical industry in 1990, an industry he served with high distinction for the remainder of his professional career.

I always viewed Irving Fox as a superstar throughout the 20 years we worked together in academia as well as the following 30 years as he progressed in the pharmaceutical industry.

William N Kelley, MD
Professor of Medicine, University of Pennsylvania.

THE
Flashing
LIGHT

A MEDICAL MYSTERY MEMOIR

THE *Flashing* LIGHT

A MEDICAL MYSTERY MEMOIR

IRVING H. FOX

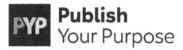

Publish Your Purpose
141 Weston Street, #155
Hartford, CT, 06141

The opinions expressed by the Author are not necessarily those held by Publish Your Purpose.

Ordering Information: Quantity sales and special discounts are available on quantity purchases by corporations, associations, and others. For details, contact the publisher at hello@publishyourpurpose.com.

Edited by: Michael Levin, Nancy Graham-Tillman

Printed in the United States of America.

ISBN: 979-8-88797-008-0 (hardcover)
ISBN: 979-8-88797-007-3 (paperback)
ISBN: 979-8-88797-009-7 (ebook)

Library of Congress Control Number: 2022921264
First edition, April 2023

Publish Your Purpose is a hybrid publisher of nonfiction books. Our mission is to elevate the voices often excluded from traditional publishing. We intentionally seek out authors and storytellers with diverse backgrounds, life experiences, and unique perspectives to publish books that will make an impact in the world. Do you have a book idea you would like us to consider publishing? Please visit PublishYourPurpose.com for more information.

This book is to inspire hope of recovery in anyone experiencing a calamitous personal event.

Contents

Foreword

Irving Fox, a long-standing friend, called me in the spring of 2020 and told me that he had decided to write about the mysterious and devastating neuropsychiatric illness he had more than fifty years ago. At the time of his illness, we were both medical residents at the Royal Victoria Hospital, a McGill University teaching hospital. Although Irving was always curious about what had happened to him, his interest was rekindled and precipitated by the discovery of his old medical files and notes he wrote during his illness that described bizarre events.

When he was ill, he was not in a position to appreciate what was happening, so he decided to begin by interviewing his friends and family for their recollections. By piecing together the stories from each person's memory, Irving hoped to gain enough information to understand more about the events that had unfolded. He planned to supplement these personal recollections with physician and nurse notes and hospital records. His illness occurred during a time before CT scans were widely available in Canada, MRIs were just being introduced, and hospital records were not computerized. Nonetheless, his medical notes, particularly those from nurses, became available when he finally received copies of his medical records from the Montreal Neurological Hospital and the Allan Memorial Institute. They were remarkably preserved after more than fifty years.

Irving and I have been friends for a long time. We met as members of the newly established McGill University seven-year medical course sometime between 1960 and 1962. This new program offered the opportunity to earn a Bachelor of Science degree and an MD, CM (McGill's Doctor of Medicine degree) in seven years instead of the usual four years spent earning an undergraduate bachelor's degree and an additional four years in medical school. During the program's third year, we decided to work together during the histology course. We developed our friendship by meeting at each other's homes in Montreal on Sunday mornings with our microscopes and slides of normal human tissues. We thought that by working together we could more efficiently assimilate the tremendous course material.

Our work with microscopes and slides carried over into our human pathology course during the program's fourth year when we studied and quizzed each other about identifying and understanding human disease from tissue samples. Our interactions continued into our clinical rotations in the form of developing index cards to help learn differential diagnoses of human signs and symptoms that patients present with. For example, if a patient had chest pain, we created a list of various diseases to consider as causes of this symptom. As it turned out, our studies together were rewarded upon graduation when we were jointly awarded the J. Francis Williams Prize in Medicine and Clinical Medicine for being first in medicine rotations.

Our personal lives also intertwined. We married good friends in the final year of medical school, and after graduation in June of 1967, both of us were accepted for a rotating internship at Montreal's renowned Royal Victoria Hospital, fondly called "The Vic." Around the time of Irving's illness, we both had advanced to Junior Assistant Resident in Medicine at The Vic.

My involvement with Irving's illness began in November 1968 when he told me about his experience with seeing a flashing blue light and the outcome of his visit to Dr. McNaughton's office the next day. To find out how he was feeling, I decided to check in with him the following Monday evening while he was on duty. What happened next was shocking and is described in detail in this book. Irving had a generalized seizure while talking to me on the phone at the nurses' station! This marked the beginning of his calamitous illness.

Irving spent the next three months in the hospital with mysterious neurological and psychiatric diseases. He spent three weeks in the Montreal Neurological Hospital and almost two months in the Allan Memorial Institute, a psychiatric hospital. He remembers very little about his psychiatric confinement. What he describes within these pages are his perspectives of the tests and treatments he underwent and the pain and suffering he endured.

My own periodic hospital visits and interactions with Irving yielded some bizarre events. I had long discussions with his wife, Gloria, who was concerned about whether Irving would ever recover from his psychotic state. I was optimistic that he would, while Gloria was profoundly worried based on her family experiences.

By the third week in February 1969, Irving was discharged to a normal life with some supervision after a vacation. This mysterious but favorable outcome was surprising but happily accepted! My hunch of his return to normalcy was validated then and during the succeeding fifty years. By the end of June 1969, Irving and I parted company as we moved to different places to pursue our personal family lives and our distinct professional ventures.

Irving is devoted to giving back. He had a highly successful career in academic medicine when, surprisingly to his faculty colleagues, he went to work in the biopharmaceutical industry because he wanted to develop novel therapies to improve the lives of thousands of patients. My own opinion is that this subconscious drive was related to his wanting to give back after recovering from his illness and "getting his life back."

Irving's life story has a key lesson for all to remember: it is possible to face horrible adversity and recover completely.

Arnold Aberman
MDCM, as Professor of Medicine Emeritus, Past Dean, Past Vice-Provost, above all at Temerty Faculty of Medicine University of Toronto
Member of Order of Canada

CHAPTER 1
Who Turned on the Light?

It's pretty common for North American men in their twenties to see bright lights in their future. I know I did. In the fall of 1968, at only twenty-four years old, I'd already been a doctor for more than a year, having graduated at the top of my class from the foremost medical school in Canada with a host of honors and awards. I was living the heady and intense life of a hospital medical resident (or house officer). Two years earlier, on an auspicious June day, I married Gloria, who remains the light of my life all these decades later.

Gloria and I both had promising careers—hers as a teacher, mine as a doctor—and we cared passionately about our respective fields. As a couple, we were blissfully happy, despite the modest lifestyle and financial challenges we faced in those salad days. We were both still students when we tied the knot. I clocked many long days and nights on the grueling, sleep-depriving rotations of hospital medical residents, but I was hard-working, energetic, and willing to pay my dues.

I'd led a somewhat sheltered life, growing up on the straight and narrow in a middle-class, Jewish family in Montreal. I think it's fair to say I was imbued with expectations of happiness and a high-achieving professional and family life. A full, robust, and healthy life.

Now, don't get the idea that I was entitled, overly self-assured, or arrogant—a word that often comes to mind, sadly, in discussions about doctors. I was none of those things. I just want you to see the picture of a rising young doctor and loving husband who believed that the stars would shine for him and the road ahead would be mostly obstacle-free. Like most people, I don't think I gave conscious thought to that assumption; it was rooted in me at some deep level.

Maybe that's what made the events that were about to unfold more surprising, even shocking—and so tough for my family and me to handle. This wasn't supposed to happen to me! But it did, and the reality is that it can happen to anyone. The mysterious symptoms and illness I developed beginning in November of 1968 threatened a serious and permanent disruption of my work and lifestyle. It threatened my very existence. And it all began with a pale, blue light.

HOW IT BEGAN: THE SCINTILLATING SCOTOMA

I don't remember what day it was.
I didn't notice what time it was.

Those lyrics begin the pop song, "More Today Than Yesterday," released by the California band The Spiral Starecase in 1969. The song's about being dazed by love, but for me it relates to the very first clue that I was about to experience a personal medical crisis I'd never dreamed possible. I don't remember what day it was. I only know it was sometime in November of 1968 when my downward health spiral began. A clear, pulsating blue light abruptly appeared in front of my eyes. When I saw it, I was sitting in a friend's parked car, minding my own business as my friend was saying goodnight to his date at her door.

The flashing blue light appeared in my field of vision in the upper-left outer quadrant. Although it seemed clear, it was very bright and I couldn't see through it. It was obstructing a big portion of my vision. What a striking experience—just incredible, coming out of nowhere like that. Closing my eyes didn't make it disappear. As I found out later, that's because the phenomenon, known as a scintillating scotoma, is caused by miscommunication in the brain. You feel like you're seeing a real object, but it's actually a fabrication of your brain.

The shimmering blue light stayed with me for about two minutes. Then it disappeared, leaving behind a sort of "after image." I couldn't see well on my left side for a little while. I had absolutely no idea what it was or why it had occurred. My friend returned to the car, and I didn't mention it. We drove off, and in the hectic demands of my everyday life, I soon forgot all about this weird, inexplicable event.

Unfortunately, the event wouldn't stay forgotten for long. On November 29, 1968, like an alien beaming down from a UFO, the flashing blue light was back. I was just leaving a colleague's office when it struck—boom—the blue coming out of the blue. Again, it lasted about two minutes. I managed to leave the office with great difficulty, even though the surroundings were familiar to me. I'd been going there frequently, working on writing up a report on a research project with my colleague Dr. Henry Gault.

In the parking lot, I just didn't feel right. I had a strange feeling on the left side of my vision, and things didn't look clear. I headed towards my car—where I thought it was, anyway—but it was nowhere in sight. After searching for a bit, I turned back around and realized my car was right there next to me. I'd walked past it because it was on my left, and, as I would soon learn, I was temporarily unable to see on that side.

It's not unusual for people in that kind of situation to normalize things in their minds. I guess I didn't know how disoriented I was, because I got in the car and started the engine. Another shock: I had absolutely no idea of how to drive out of the parking lot. Can you imagine how it felt for a twenty-four-year-old to suddenly find himself absolutely incapable of performing a routine activity he'd done so many times in the past? I began to grow anxious. Then I recalled a story I'd heard in medical school about a doctor who discovered he couldn't see on the left side of his visual field. He had a brain tumor.

Increasingly frantic, I summoned my medical training and tried a test: looking straight ahead while passing my finger in front of my eyes to the left. The finger vanished. I tested again, and with each eye, the finger would disappear from view as it moved left. Panic set in, big time. I was trembling. Nevertheless, I foolishly persuaded myself a second time that I could drive. Luckily for me and others, I was clueless as to which way to go and quickly abandoned that bonkers idea.

I screamed silently to myself, "You have a brain tumor. It's game over!" I felt nauseated and climbed out of my car, doing the finger test over and over, unable to believe this was really happening. Dr. Gault was about to depart in his own car. In a scene straight out of slapstick comedy, he saw my raised finger and thought I was signaling to him. He walked over, asking, "Can't find your car?"

"I don't feel very well," I responded, maintaining my doctor's demeanor while reporting dispassionately on the flashing light, the loss of my left visual field, and a slight headache I'd had all week. "I think I have a brain tumor." Dr. Gault escorted me back into his office, where he wiggled his fingers on both sides of my head and confirmed my findings. He decided to take me to the emergency room (ER). Just as we were leaving, my vision returned, but the mystery remained.

DIRE THOUGHTS

Physically, I was heading to the hospital with Dr. Gault. But inside my head, I was traveling to the land of fear, catastrophizing, and self-pity, coupled with perhaps a little too much medical knowledge for my own good in that particular circumstance. I sank into despair. I remembered that on the ward of the chest hospital where I was then working, three patients had died in the past ten days of lung cancer.

"Isn't it ironic that I'll soon be following them, dying of brain cancer?" I thought, taking myself step by imaginary step through the medical process, right down to picturing the surgeons operating on my brain. I told myself that even if they successfully removed the tumor, I'd be useless. "Who wants a doctor with some of his brain cut out?" By the time we arrived at the ER of Royal Victoria Hospital (RVH), I was fighting to hold back my tears.

On the ER paperwork, I reported my symptoms as a severe headache, and I sat in the ER waiting area until I could see the neurology resident. I spotted Gloria coming in the door, and a few tears trickled down my cheek. Discreetly, I brushed them aside, thinking to myself, "What a beautiful and tragic young widow my wife will be."

DOCTOR BECOMES PATIENT

Obviously, I didn't die of a brain tumor or anything else. In the coming chapters, I'll take you through a medical mystery tale of what would prove to be a months-long ordeal that began with the flashing blue light that November day in my friend's car. I had seizures and many other serious physical and psychiatric symptoms, and I wound up hospitalized in two different facilities for roughly three months beginning a few days after the ER visit.

The doctors had well-informed guesses, but they couldn't pinpoint what was causing my symptoms. They sometimes had conflicting opinions about what was wrong and how to treat it. I went through repeated tests and screening procedures, some of which were excruciating; blessedly, they have been replaced by tests that are less painful, less invasive, and more effective at investigating problems.

I'm not sure how many of my doctors thought I'd survive, much less recover fully. They deserve plenty of credit for persisting and hanging in there with me, always looking for better approaches and new solutions. Eventually, after many weeks of not remembering what day or time it was, I seemed to turn a corner. My health and mental status began improving until, miraculously, I was well enough to go home.

Soon I was feeling vastly better. As you can imagine after an affliction that severe, my wife, my parents, and I didn't really trust that I was out of the woods. But I guess we'd learned some lessons about life's fragility and brevity, because we returned to our pre-illness routines in remarkably speedy fashion with renewed vigor.

Within a short time of my final discharge, we were completely immersed in numerous significant life changes that came down the pike in rapid succession. Vacations, illnesses of other family members, fellowships, job changes, relocation from Canada to North Carolina, and Gloria's pregnancy took our minds away from my sickness as well as our fears that it might recur. (It did not!)

Naturally, I never forgot about the most traumatic health event of my life, but I did push it aside, stowing the memory in the back of my brain like a funky old lamp tucked away in the attic. It wasn't until another traumatic health event—a global one in 2020—that I found the time to start exploring my personal medical history.

PANDEMIC PARALLELS

After I retired from my second career in pharmaceutical research, I launched a consulting business. Then the COVID-19 pandemic took hold in the winter of 2020. We all quickly became familiar with terms such as social distancing, lockdowns, droplets, aerosol, Zoom, Instacart, PPE, and remote learning. We scoured the internet for toilet paper and hand sanitizer. Airlines slashed flights. Restaurants closed their dining rooms, retooling for takeout and delivery only. Sporting events and other public entertainment venues shut down. Many retail businesses that were forced to close during the strictest lockdown periods never opened their doors again.

With travel being risky and so many other challenges, my consulting business became a victim of the pandemic. Gloria always said I was a workaholic and what she called a "studyholic." I thrive on working and keeping busy. Once the pandemic hit, I had entirely too much time on my hands. More and more, I found myself thinking back to my mysterious illness, drawn to learn more about this dramatic, life-altering period. Soon, I decided to tackle it as a research project, which resulted in writing this book.

Did the COVID-19 pandemic prompt my decision to look into my old health condition? Possibly, though it wasn't as strong a motivator as stumbling into all that free time. I certainly don't mean to amplify my own tiny-scale personal health crisis by comparing it with the horrible impact and magnitude of a pandemic that has killed millions of people. Still, there are a number of parallels between the two that may have subtly influenced me to launch this project.

For one thing, both my illness and COVID carry many unknowns and mysteries. The virus that causes COVID, SARS-CoV-2, was known at first as a novel coronavirus because it was believed to be new to the world. Initially, little to nothing was known about its origin, how it spread around the world, how it infected people, how symptoms would manifest in different people, or what treatments and prevention methods might be effective. Likewise, there was quite a bit about the origin, course, symptoms, and treatment of my illness that were unknown and based only on best guesses. Even today, after my exploration, all I know about my own diagnosis amounts to nothing more than a solid, educated guess.

In addition, both COVID and my condition had the potential to be gravely serious illnesses with lethal outcomes. Both also carried the possibility of lingering, long-term effects, such as those associated with long COVID. In my case, doctors simply couldn't be certain whether I'd have lasting problems or disabilities if I were fortunate enough to recover from the acute part of the illness.

The third parallel is that my illness and COVID were both major disruptors. From lockdowns and supply chain problems to school closures and the growth of the fact-denying anti-vaccine movement, COVID has turned our lives upside down. So too, though to a vastly smaller degree, did my medical mystery rattle my life. Had things gone ever-so-slightly differently, it could easily have derailed my medical career. As for Gloria and our families and friends, many were negatively impacted or put their lives on hold as everyone visited, supported, cried, and prayed.

METHODOLOGY FOR LEARNING THE HISTORY OF MY MYSTERY

For much of the duration of my illness, I was nearly incapacitated and usually heavily medicated. My personal memory of those months is almost a blank. Along with that, the passage of more than half a century has caused most of the memories I did have to fade. I have, however, gathered multiple sources of information and documentation, allowing me to piece together a reliable picture of what was happening.

My exploration began with a decrepit, musty-smelling old cardboard box in the basement of my home here in Wellesley, Massachusetts. For some reason, instead of framing all my diplomas and awards and hanging them on a wall, I had stashed them—even my med school diploma—in that box, in their original scrolls and wrappings. From among all those relics and mementos, I pulled out the ratty old manila folder I was seeking.

In it I found my notes, handwritten in a diary bearing the name of the Montreal Neurological Hospital (MNH), where I'd been admitted twice in December of 1968 before being transferred for a two-month stay at the Allan Memorial Institute (AMI), a psychiatric hospital. The yellowed pages of the diary were stiffening but hadn't yet started to crumble, and the writing was legible. (Well, legible at least to me since I possess the notoriously inscrutable handwriting of a doctor. And my scrawl was even worse thanks to my illness and distraught state of mind.)

As I read my notes, my mind wandered back to that calamitous period more than fifty years earlier. Was that really me, Irving Fox? It was a peculiar feeling. I'd done a good job burying these memories in the recesses of my brain. But now my desire to find out what actually happened to me grew more intense. I embarked on an eight-month journey to rediscover my past.

I began by methodically dictating the notes into a digital recorder for later transcription by Adam Spielman, my teenage grandson, who was eager to earn some extra cash for the job. He proved to be an enormous help, teaching me how to use computer technology and Google Docs more efficiently so that we could collaborate remotely from our different locations. The tedious work had the wonderful fringe benefit of strengthening the bond between Adam and me, bringing us closer together during the time of pandemic separations. Though only sixteen, he offered me some valuable input on how to structure this book.

The notes were more like personal reflections than medical records. And they were written almost exclusively during that first month of my illness in December of 1968. To supplement the information, I began recording interviews with friends and family who knew me back then, trying to elicit more details that might fill in some of the blanks. Unfortunately, most of the medical providers who had treated me and might have had insights on my case had passed away or didn't recall details from all those years ago. I realized the materials I had thus far collected were insufficient, so I set out to acquire my fifty-two-year-old medical records. I had no idea whether they could be located or would even be legible. But I was determined to try.

It took four months and the patience of Job before hard copies of my pristinely preserved medical records arrived via old-fashioned snail mail. They included doctors' notes and diagnoses, test results, bedside nursing notes, and comprehensive discharge summaries, sent to me by McGill University Health Center and MNH. These documents were complete and impressively displayed the high-quality medical practice at McGill Medical School's teaching hospitals in the late 1960s.

Finally, I had the facts I needed to reconstruct my long-ago health saga. And although I was interested in filling gaps for personal reasons, this was not really an exercise in idle curiosity. Medicine and science have advanced at lightning speed over the last fifty years, but the more we learn, the more we realize how much is still unknown.

Because I had so many memory lapses from the time, I was able to step back—to review the materials from my own medical story almost as if I were an outside doctor brought in to consult. With only a tad of bias, I can frankly say this was a fascinating case, filled with diagnostic and treatment question marks, bizarre physical and psychiatric symptoms, conflicts of medical opinion, and a miraculous recovery that happened almost as mysteriously as the whole thing started.

In exploring this decades-old puzzle, I found insights, understanding, and approaches to perplexing medical cases that are still applicable today, even with all our scientific advancements. I offer my story and the results of my investigation in the hope that others who are facing complex and seemingly unfathomable health crises will find tools and information to apply for the benefit of themselves or their loved ones.

CHAPTER 2
Wellesley, Massachusetts, Spring, 2020

The spring of 2020 found Gloria and me cooped up in our home in Wellesley, Massachusetts. COVID-19 had hit hard in the US. The earliest and worst US outbreak caused utter devastation in New York City, where the first case was reported on March 1, 2020. Within a week, the governor declared a state of emergency. By mid-March, two people in New York had died of COVID. Before three months had passed, the death toll exploded into the tens of thousands.

COVID-19 had slammed into New York like a colossal hurricane and tornado combined. It was shocking. It was fearsome. It was hard to believe. If you got the disease, it was often physically traumatizing. If you didn't, even if you didn't live in New York or another outbreak center, it could be mentally traumatizing.

From Wellesley, just a few hours away, we watched television coverage of the unfolding New York crisis in abject horror. With the city under strict lockdown, the normally bustling streets and subways became ghost towns. Lines of ambulances backed up for blocks outside overflowing hospitals, waiting hours on end to find beds for their desperately ill patients who lay there coughing, in pain, and struggling to breathe. News stories and images that emerged from inside hospitals offered grizzly depictions of conditions for patients and staff. Deprived of adequate protective equipment, medical personnel were falling ill and dying in alarming numbers.

After bodies were found in an unrefrigerated U-Haul truck outside a backlogged funeral home in Brooklyn, authorities sent in a fleet of refrigerated tractor trailers, retooled as makeshift morgues. A year later, several hundred corpses remained in those trucks in South Brooklyn. Thousands of victims were buried in unadorned pine caskets in a mass graveyard on Hart Island, just off the Bronx between New York and Long Island.

The US Centers for Disease Control and Prevention says the "crude fatality rate" from COVID in New York in the early months was 9.2 percent of those infected, a stunningly high percentage. Of those hospitalized, more than 32 percent lost their lives.[1] People were dying at home, too, and the military was deployed to neighborhoods to collect victims' bodies. Between March and May, New York City's COVID death toll was estimated at more than thirty thousand.

New York was the original US epicenter for COVID in the first half of 2020, but it didn't take long for the wily virus to rampage its way around the country. The delivery of a safe, effective, and widely available COVID vaccine was nearly a year in the future, though in historical perspective,

---

[1.] Thompson CN, Baumgartner J, Pichardo C, et al. COVID-19 Outbreak — New York City, February 29–June 1, 2020. MMWR Morbidity and Mortality Weekly Report 69 (November 20, 2020): 1725–1729, http://dx.doi.org/10.15585/mmwr.mm6946a2external icon.

the vaccines were researched, developed, and produced with remarkable speed. As someone who spent a couple dozen years in drug research and development, I think the COVID-19 vaccine development process was—and is—an absolutely tremendous accomplishment.

Despite the enormous skill and dedication of doctors, nurses, and other medical and support staff, treatment was essentially guesswork. It was solid, science-based, and experience-based, though that experience was with other diseases, not COVID-19. In no way am I criticizing the methods. Medical providers delivered the best care possible under unimaginably difficult circumstances. I'm using the term "guesswork" simply to emphasize how much about this novel coronavirus and its impact on humans was a mystery to us.

Extensive testing might have slowed down COVID's spread, but for a variety of reasons, rollout of an early nation-wide testing program never occurred. Protective gear was scarce. We didn't know or didn't implement optimal practices for preventing transmission. We weren't even sure when and how the virus was transmissible. We didn't have a vaccine, and we didn't know the best therapies. We didn't know about long COVID or about the risks for people who had COVID after they had recovered from acute COVID.

In short, despite the advanced and near-miraculous state of modern medicine, the COVID-19 knowledge base was pretty much a blank slate in those first weeks and months. And while we know vastly more today and have a greatly improved arsenal for prevention, testing, and treatment, it's important to remember that expertise is expanding while the virus is mutating and changing the manner in which it causes disease. So, we're still living in a world of unknowns, where today's best practice may become outdated tomorrow.

Unfortunately, the field of medicine is anything but cut and dried. As a culture, many Americans carry underlying assumptions about the magic-bullet nature of medical care. Take a pill, get better. It's funny in a way. Given the lightning-fast pace of technological advancement in the last hundred years, you'd think we'd have learned to better tolerate change and uncertainty. But when it comes to personal health outcomes, such tolerance is uncommon. As is patience.

While researchers and doctors were furiously working to fill the COVID blank slate with credible, verifiable facts and practical information, another force was countering their efforts. Misinformation, mistrust, misconceptions, downright lies, and conspiracy theories were spreading on the web like another pandemic. Social media and instantaneous access to unvetted videos on sites such as YouTube played an outsized role in the growth of misinformation. People with little to no foundation for understanding such a complex disease "did their own research" and came away with a set of intractable, emotionally based beliefs about COVID that were vastly distorted and, quite frankly, detached from reality. Much of this was harmful. We knew little in those early days, but there were things we were learning, quickly. Hydroxychloroquine was promptly shown to have no benefit in treating or preventing COVID. Drinking bleach was dangerous and not remotely effective, while wearing well-fitting masks offered strong protection. These were irrefutable facts that millions of people chose not to believe.

There's nothing new about mistrust, medical misinformation, and snake-oil hype. What's new is that most of us now hold in our hands a device that allows worldwide communication and unlimited split-second access to an overwhelming volume of information. There are no filters to distinguish truth from falsehood, reality from fantasy, or authentically informative materials from manipulative ones produced by those with ulterior motives. Into this bizarre digital milieu arose a disease that became the worst pandemic in a century—since the 1918 Spanish flu pandemic that was believed to have killed fifty million people. COVID-19 was born into a strange new world.

ALIEN LANDSCAPE

Though there was a mountain of unknowns, I had the medical training to understand more than most people about the COVID public health crisis. From the standpoint of our personal health, I knew one thing with 100 percent certainty: due to our age, Gloria and I were at high risk of severe symptoms, hospitalization, and death if we caught COVID-19. I have rheumatoid arthritis, an autoimmune disease that further enhances my risk level together with my immune inhibitory treatment with methotrexate.

Well, I felt I'd already done more than my share of time in a hospital bed, thank you. We said a resounding "No!" to the prospect of catching COVID. We didn't want to spend possibly our final weeks or months in isolation, talking with our loved ones only over a computer screen, suffering miserably, and maybe getting intubated and hooked up to ventilators. We stayed home. When vaccines became available, we got them. We took all the precautions we could, based on the best available knowledge. When that knowledge changed, we adapted our practices as necessary. We were lucky to have each other for comfort and companionship. Many people had to face the fear and isolation of COVID all alone.

As I write this, the latest dominant coronavirus mutation is a subvariant of the Omicron variant that's known as BA.5. This mutation seems to have increased both the infectiousness of the disease and its ability to "escape" or get by the body's protective antibody response that comes from vaccination and/or previous infection. Researchers are now trying to anticipate the likely viral mutation process, looking ahead to creating new vaccines that last longer and offer more universal protection against a variety of SARS-CoV-2 mutations.

I hold out a confident hope that before too long, researchers will bring us new vaccines and therapeutics (treatments) to get and maintain a handle on COVID-19. Nevertheless, this virus has proven to be anything but static, and complacency is dangerous. We've come a long, long way since the pandemic's onset, but many uncertainties remain.

As I observed the disturbing developments from my perch at home in Wellesley in the spring of 2020, I had the eerie experience of feeling like I'd been dropped into an alien landscape. Or, perhaps, that the alien landscape had been dropped into the middle of my established world. Honestly, it was a little weird, like a twilight zone. The feelings of strangeness may have been amplified by the loss of my consulting business and this workaholic's sudden confinement to home after decades of toiling away, late into the night, on multiple jobs and projects simultaneously.

It was in this mood of strangeness—separated from my lifelong routines and habits—that I first pulled out that old folder containing my personal notes of my mysterious illness of 1968–1969. All but one was written during the first month, in December of 1968, and they comprised an odd collection of writings. One day, I'd wax poetic about the more mundane aspects of having my temperature taken rectally when I was hospitalized. Another day, I'd take a look at overarching philosophical questions of meaning and purpose. And then, in a different entry, I'd seem to have my doctor's hat on as I described a procedure I'd undergone.

How curious! I didn't recognize myself in those writings. My memories of the period were so vague, diluted by time and the business of living a full life. Have you ever leafed through an old photo album and had it stir up long-dormant recollections, maybe of people and events in that earlier part of your life? I was sort of hoping that reading these diary entries might kick loose some of the memories. Instead, it was more like opening the old album to find the pictures had faded and peeled, making it difficult to identify people and places.

Incomplete though the picture was, I found my personal notes fascinating all these years later. It spurred me to do additional research and seek out my medical records. I felt compelled to find out more about what had happened. I wanted to understand the events that transpired using my present medical expertise and experience. Speaking candidly, I also wanted to get a closer, deeper, and more contextual look at this young man—the former me—who had gone through so much during this twilight zone period.

How had my ordeal influenced my future life and career? And how had my earlier life shaped the young man who'd endured this extraordinary medical and psychiatric crisis? In a sense, in 2020, I conducted a metaphorical archeological dig into my own past, examining who I was and what events befell me leading up to my mysterious illness and in its immediate aftermath. I pondered my early life story for any more context I might discover. I'll share that with you in the next chapter, as a backdrop to provide a more complete portrait of me before I began my three-month-long dance with illness and mortality.

CHAPTER 3
Kit Fox

I've described the weird, altered-reality qualities the world seemed to take on during two major health-related events in my life: the mystery illness that struck shortly before I turned twenty-five late in 1968 and the COVID-19 pandemic that began in 2020.

Reflecting on these periods, I realized there was a third strange and distorted era in my life, one of which I have no memories. This was a horrific time that reshaped the world, upending hundreds of millions of lives while spreading fear, uncertainty, suffering, and death across the globe: I was born in the middle of World War II. My birthday on December 7, 1943, came on the second anniversary of Japan's devastating surprise attack on the Pearl Harbor naval base in Hawaii. The bombing of Pearl Harbor propelled the US to enter the war on the side of the Allies—against Japan, Germany, and Italy.

Canada was actually the first country in the Western Hemisphere to declare war on Japan, doing so within hours of Pearl Harbor. Canada had entered the European part of the war more than two years earlier than the US. Canada declared war on Nazi Germany in September of 1939, about a week after German Chancellor Adolf Hitler sent his troops to invade Poland.

The war had a huge impact on Canada. Over the six years until the defeat of the Axis countries, more than a million Canadians served in the military, quite a substantial percentage for a nation that then had fewer than twelve million people. Canadians participated in all theatres of operation, although much of the country's efforts were concentrated in Italy—first against Benito Mussolini's regime, then fighting to defeat the Germans in Italy. More than forty-two thousand Canadians died in the war, with another fifty-five thousand wounded. The losses were deeply felt.

Shifting to a wartime economy quashed the Great Depression in Canada, thanks to a massive ramping-up of production in the areas of weapons manufacturing, war-related industries, and food and agriculture. But most of the extra production of food and materials went to supply the overseas campaigns, as well as to the citizens of our mother country, Great Britain. The German assaults on Britain's land and water had cut off the island, causing dire shortages, adversity, and great suffering for the British.

At home, Canadians like my parents sacrificed for the greater good and learned to live in a new reality. Despite the hardship, Canadians were generally eager to do whatever they could to help defend our democratic freedoms and defeat tyranny. Citizens received ration books containing coupons that allowed them to wait in long lines to buy piddling amounts of common foods. Among other items, meat, sugar, butter, cheese, coffee, tea, and alcohol were strictly rationed. Fresh fruit, ice cream, and desserts were almost unseen during the war. When they could, people hunted and fished, picked wild berries, grew "victory gardens," and learned to can, pickle, and preserve. Folks made do with potatoes and turnips—not exactly the top palate pleasers. Fuel was rationed, and everyday items were also in short supply. Paper was difficult to find. Even clothing wasn't readily available, as wool and other fabrics were needed to make uniforms, parachutes, and related gear. I was born into a world of scarcity, sacrifice, and struggle.

It was also a world of fear and worry. Today's intensely hostile social and political environment, along with the pandemic and the effects of climate change, has created enormous anxiety about the future. As disturbing as it is, today's malaise in the US offers only a limited sense of the overwhelming sentiment ordinary people felt during the war—which was literally a world war, involving all seven continents in one way or another.

For Jewish families such as ours, it's fair to say the anxiety was amplified many times over. Inconceivable atrocities were being committed against the Jews in the cause of genocide. Allied victory was not assured. Outside of the German-occupied countries, Jews worried that the Nazis might prevail and expand the Holocaust across increasingly more falling borders. Rationing beef was one thing. Having to move your family into a hidden room or flee a country for your lives was quite another.

FAMILY ROOTS

Having already made it through the ordeal of the Great Depression, my parents and grandparents adapted once again to a new situation, this time to the challenges of living on a war footing in Montreal. They managed to function as normally as possible amidst the supremely abnormal. And much to their credit, my parents were able to provide comfort and security for me and my two younger siblings, both during the war and in its aftermath. Given the brutal nature of the war, and the fact that the persecution and murder of

Jews had long been part of my family's history, this was no small accomplishment.

My parents were Nathan Fox and Phyllis (Fanny) Fox, née Maron. Both were second-generation Canadians, from families of Jewish descent through many generations. They both grew up in Outremont, a beautiful, picturesque, and affluent borough in Montreal, where the late Prime Minister Pierre Trudeau was born and raised. (He was the father of current Prime Minister Justin Trudeau.) In Outremont, my parents were contemporaries of the famous novelist Mordechai Richler, whose many books include *The Apprenticeship of Duddy Kravitz*.

Although my parents shared a few cultural similarities, their courtship and marriage were rather unlikely, given that their fathers held such starkly divergent sociopolitical views. Solomon Fox, my grandfather, was a Russian-born farm boy who immigrated to Canada in 1912 at about age nineteen. He probably escaped by the skin of his teeth—a few short years before the Russian Revolution that ushered in the Communist era and brought Vladimir Lenin to power as the first leader of Soviet Russia and then the Soviet Union. When he came to Canada, Solomon carried a fierce hatred of anything Russian or Communist. Russia and neighboring East European lands had been, to say the least, inhospitable places to be Jewish. Solomon's father, my great-grandfather, had been murdered by Cossacks, a semi-nomadic ethnic group who were Christian Orthodox. The Cossacks were known for carrying out many horrendous, savage attacks on Jewish villages, in which they would loot, rape, and massacre, then expel any Jews who survived. In the nineteenth and twentieth centuries, these riotous, violent attacks became known as *pogroms.*

You can see why Solomon continued to harbor ill will towards all things Russian when he arrived in Canada. Determined to have a better life with financial security, he became a wholesale butcher and dabbled in real estate, eventually buying and operating a number of apartment buildings. When the stock market crashed in 1929, he lost $75,000—a huge amount of money in those days. Solomon locked himself in a room for three days, but he eventually recovered from his despair.

By contrast, my mother's father, Louis Maron, had emigrated from Minsk, which was then controlled by the Russian Empire and today is part of Belarus. Louis worked in a machine shop for the Canadian National Railway and was a loyal union member. He was also a member of the Canadian Communist Party, thus a polar opposite of the eager capitalist Solomon Fox. In those days, parents had a lot more say about their children's marital choices than they do today. Still, Nathan and Fanny somehow found each other, cast off the biases of their fathers, and got married.

My two grandmothers were Rachel Fox and Molly Maron. Molly was a typical Jewish bubbie (from the Yiddish word *bubbe*, meaning grandmother.) She was warm, physically affectionate, and always a wonderful and welcoming hostess. In my memory, I see her as four feet tall and four feet wide. My god, what an incredible cook she was! I may not remember anything about the two months I spent in a psych hospital, but I can still taste my grandmother Molly's luscious cooking.

Rachel Fox, née Cohen, was as different from Molly as Solomon was from Louis. Actually, she broke the stereotypes of wives, mothers, and grandmothers of the time. Unlike my three other grandparents, Rachel came from Leeds, England, not Eastern Europe. And she didn't know how to cook. Solomon, who was eight years her senior, did all the cooking and absolutely doted on her. She called him "Dad." Rachel had a good education and wanted that for her son.

When Rachel insisted that my father attend college rather than follow Solomon into the meat business as a butcher, she got her way. Hoping to become a doctor, Nathan applied to McGill—my eventual medical school alma mater. In the early 1940s, McGill had a cap on the number of Jewish students it would enroll, thus my father was rejected on the basis of his religion. Persistent, he instead started med school at the University of Montreal. But it was not in the cards. The school was conducted in French, which my father didn't speak, read, or write. He found the program too difficult because of this and, after a week, switched to a pharmacy major. That proved to be the ticket. Nathan earned a degree in pharmacy and owned and ran a drug store after graduation. He later became the chief pharmacist at RVH in Montreal.

BOYHOOD

My mother had not yet turned twenty when she gave birth to me at RVH during a raging December snowstorm in 1943. We lived in a western part of Montreal for a few years, then moved to the city of Côte St. Luc, also on the island of Montreal in the province of Quebec. My brother Allan came along eighteen months after me, and my sister Rosanne is four years younger than me. Growing up, I remember our home being like Grand Central Station, teeming with friends coming and going, always snacking on food from my mother's well-stocked pantry. On Sundays, we'd visit grandparents and enjoy the company of our cousins, aunts, and uncles.

I wasn't very good at organized team sports and didn't play them much as a young child. I didn't have much time, anyway, since I attended Hebrew school at Shaare Zion Beth-El Congregation five days a week. I think my Jewish education served as an important counterbalance to my "regular" education, which was at the Protestant School Board of Greater Montreal. Why would a Jewish boy attend a Protestant school? There was no separation of church and state in 1950s Montreal. Most Jewish families chose to send their kids to Protestant rather than Catholic schools. That's just the way things were. Every morning I'd go to school, salute the flag, say the Lord's Prayer, read from the New Testament, and sing hymns such as "Onward Christian Soldier." I played a shepherd in a school Christmas pageant and learned to love Christmas music and caroling. Then, every day after school, off I'd go to learn Hebrew and study Torah for ninety minutes, reinforcing my Jewish identity.

No, my head did not explode. It was a normalized way of life for us. Attending a Christian school didn't detract from my Jewish practice in the slightest. My exposure to Christianity broadened my horizons and has been helpful at times throughout my life. When I became a bar mitzvah at thirteen, my family threw a terrific celebration to honor the occasion. I remained observant for another year or two, until I found myself questioning the existence of God. That's when I became agnostic, something that lasted only until my first child was born and I rediscovered my relationship with the divine.

My post-bar-mitzvah teenage years were a great deal of fun, very social, and, once again, pretty normal and uneventful. Without Hebrew school to attend, I had more time for biking, skating, and playing hockey and baseball informally with my friends. I joined the local B'nai B'rith Jewish youth group and took part in their activities. Starting around age thirteen, I dated a series of girls, but it never got any more serious than slow dancing or an occasional game of Spin the Bottle. Sometimes my friends and

I would go to an amusement park or take the streetcar to bustling downtown Montreal.

THE MEDICAL TRACK

I studied hard in high school and did quite well, pursuing a course called engineering that basically emphasized math and physics. At that time, I hoped to become a physicist. But during my final high school year, I heard about a seven-year medical program at McGill that really grabbed my interest. It was like college and med school combined. I could start intense medical studies in year four, earn a Bachelor of Science degree after year five, and get an MD at the end of year seven. I decided to apply and was happy to be accepted. At that time, I wasn't aware of the ridiculous Jewish quota, which remained in place until the late 1960s.

I mentioned earlier that when I had my first flashing blue light episode, I was only twenty-four and had already been a doctor for more than a year. That may seem quite young to Americans. In 1950s Canada, high school ended after eleventh grade. Having a December birthday, I had started school early. That's why I entered university in September of 1960 at only sixteen, knowing that if all went well, I could be a physician by age twenty-three. I knew it would be tough going, but I felt ready, willing, and able. My confidence was only slightly shaken during McGill orientation, when a speaker instructed us to "Look to your left. Look to your right. One of you three will not be here next year." That motivated me to buckle down and take my education seriously.

BITTEN BY THE LOVE BUG:
A VERY HEALTHY INFECTION

At McGill, I took the prerequisite courses that were must-haves for the medical program. But mostly I chose a diversity of classes that were unrelated to medicine, studying everything from music appreciation to philosophy to calculus. My course load was still heavily weighted towards my strengths and interests in science and math. I found the humanities classes more challenging.

After my first year in the McGill program, in the summer of 1961, I was a "mature college man" on a fast track to becoming what I hoped would be a physician researcher. But at only seventeen, I was still drawn to youthful pastimes. I got a job as a counselor at a Jewish federation summer camp located in the Laurentian Mountains northwest of Montreal. Camp Wooden Acres was a relatively small camp, situated on the pristine, pine-encircled Lac-de-la-Montagne in Saint-Adolphe-d'Howard, Quebec.

In this scenic mountain setting, I met a fifteen-year-old counselor-in-training named Gloria Godine. I admit I found her more beautiful and interesting than the majestic scenery all around us. Back home after camp, with encouragement from my friend Lenny Diamond, I finally worked up the nerve to overcome my apprehension and ask Gloria out on a date. My heart leapt when she accepted! That first date led to a five-year courtship followed by an enduring and happy marriage. You can forget everything else you read in this book about some of the earth-shaking events of my life and career. Marrying Gloria was the best decision I ever made and had the most profound and wonderful impact on my life.

As we got engaged, I offered Gloria an exit door, explaining that although I was in med school my plan was to become a medical researcher, a career with limited earning potential. Happily, she hung in with me and we soon began our life's journey together as husband and wife. Solomon Fox, whom I called Zayde (Yiddish for Grandpa), gave me a gift of $4,000. Doesn't sound like much now, but in the mid-1960s it was a nice cushion, especially for a pair of newlyweds who were both still in school.

MARRIAGE, MED SCHOOL, AND THE OPEN ROAD

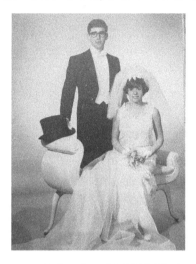

Irving and Gloria were married on June 21, 1966. Gloria was 20 years old and had just received her Bachelor of Arts degree from McGill University. Irving was 22 years old and had just completed his third year of Medical School.

Gloria and I were married in a formal wedding at her Orthodox synagogue, Congregation Beth Ora, in the borough of Saint Laurent where she grew up. Light is a recurring theme in my story, and it emerged again at our nuptials. Beth Ora means "House of Light," and we were married on the summer solstice—the longest day of the year—on June 21, 1966. It was a blissful, momentous occasion for us. Little did we know that just a couple of years later, Gloria's love and light would help steer me through the dark, somber period of my illness and hospitalization.

That was the summer before my last year of medical school. Gloria had just graduated from college and, in the fall, would head to a teacher's college for a one-year certification program. While our lives seemed unremarkable in many ways, our honeymoon was anything but conventional.

A typical honeymoon for many of our friends at the time would be to fly off to a Caribbean resort for a week and sip piña coladas on a tropical beach. Instead of that, we prepared for a cross-continental adventure built around a six-week clinical clerkship in medicine that I'd landed at Moffitt Hospital in San Francisco. My father loaned me his second car, a General Motors Acadian. We packed it up with our belongings, a tent, and sleeping bags and hit the road. We planned two weeks of travel in each direction, so we'd be gone for about ten weeks.

Westbound, we took the Trans-Canada Highway from Montreal to Vancouver, then made a left to enter the US and drive south through Washington, Oregon, and finally Northern California and San Francisco. The trip was about four thousand miles. We took our time, sightseeing along the way. As newlyweds and students we needed to pinch pennies, so we camped out—most of the time, anyway. I think Gloria would sometimes get a little weary of the camping conditions, and on those days we'd find a motel with a comfortable bed and nice, hot shower.

We saw some utterly magnificent scenery and had many unique experiences. In 1966, the portion of the Trans-Canada Highway above Lake Superior was still an unpaved dirt road. That was unexpected and forced us to drive more slowly and cautiously. We had so much fun driving, chatting, stopping when we wished, looking in awe at the countryside, and giggling together about making love in a tent. We came across a town in Ontario called Wawa and laughed uproariously at the name. We couldn't resist a souvenir, and the town of Wawa was relieved of one of its city signs.

Banff and Lake Louise in Alberta, Canada, were simply breathtaking, though that stop was a tad diminished by a rookie camping error. We put a ground sheet under the tent because the land seemed moist. I guess it rained as we slept, as we were awakened during the night with our legs soaked in a puddle of chilly water that had accumulated under the tent and was trapped by the ground sheet. We spent half the day recovering from the mess, warming and drying ourselves, figuring out how to air out the tent, and scouting a laundromat to run the sleeping bags through the dryer.

SAN FRANCISCO: SUMMER, 1966

Simultaneously weary and giddy from our adventures, Gloria and I crossed the Golden Gate Bridge into San Francisco after about ten days on the road. We settled into an apartment that I'd sublet from a University of California medical student who was away for the summer. It was located atop one of San Francisco's many hills, conveniently located near the UC San Francisco Medical Center. Each morning, I'd walk down the hill to Moffitt Hospital through the cool morning mist, breathing in the scent of eucalyptus, which was somehow sharp, pungent, minty, and sweet, all at the same time. That particular sense memory remains fixed in my mind as definitive of San Francisco.

The clerkship turned out to be a valuable one, with fascinating patients to evaluate and attending physicians who were fantastic clinical teachers. I learned a great deal. I also took some time to explore the school's highly regarded clinical pharmacology fellowship program for possible postgraduate training.

Life in the little hilltop apartment was our first substantial experience living together as a couple, and we thoroughly enjoyed it. Well, OK, there were some bumps, such as the time Gloria frantically phoned me at work, weeping. Like something out of an episode of *I Love Lucy*, the Mixmaster had somehow spewed mashed potatoes all over the walls and ceiling of our apartment kitchen.

Northern California is a beautiful, ecologically diverse area, with much to see and do. Gloria and I took full advantage of my days off, visiting places such as Carmel, Big Sur, Lake Tahoe, and Stinson Beach. We saw the beautiful redwood trees that are unique to the region. Besides being an urban community, the city of San Francisco is a tourist mecca that kept us quite busy. We rode the cable cars and explored North Beach, Chinatown, Golden Gate Park, and more.

One area we drove by but never stopped at was the Haight-Ashbury district, which was then the heart of the counterculture movement. Dressed in loose, flowing clothes and with flowers weaved into their long, natural hair, hippies, flower children, peaceniks, and political activists flocked to San Francisco from all over the country. These young folks came to protest injustice and the war in Vietnam, demand equality and civil rights for all, and partake in the free love, rock and roll, psychedelic drugs, social discourse, and open-minded communities that were radically altering the culture in the 1960s.

Coming from our sheltered, suburban, Jewish communities in Montreal, Gloria and I had had no exposure to the hippie culture—and frankly, we didn't want any. As Gloria says, "It didn't interest us. We were goodie-goodies, straight and narrow. That just wasn't our scene. We wouldn't go anywhere near those people." But other than that, Gloria very much liked San Francisco and the Bay Area. Two years later, she was disappointed when we didn't move there for the pharmacology fellowship and went instead to Durham, North Carolina.

HOMEWARD BOUND

My clerkship complete, another year of school awaited us both in Montreal. We made sure we'd gotten all the mashed potatoes off the walls, packed up the Acadian, and hit the road once more. Eager to explore more of the US, we headed south before turning back towards the Canadian border. We drove down to Southern California and visited Los Angeles and Disneyland. Then we headed east, through the high desert of California, and into Las Vegas, Nevada. It was brutally hot, and our car was not air conditioned. But somehow, we felt that driving across the desert in 100+ degree heat with brittle, dry winds blowing through our wide-open windows was a rich part of our travel experience.

Speaking of richness, we didn't hit the jackpot in Las Vegas. We didn't actually risk anything gambling. In fact, Gloria got kicked out of the Caesar's Palace casino. She was not yet twenty-one and they were extremely strict. We spent the night in Las Vegas, though, and caught a great show. From there, it was on to see the spectacular Grand Canyon in Arizona. Worn down a little from the overbearing climate, we were refreshed by a visit to Phoenix, where relatives put us up in a nice, air-conditioned hotel and treated us like royalty.

We planned the rest of our route home through several US national parks: Bryce Canyon in Utah, Yellowstone and Grand Teton in Wyoming, and Mount Rushmore in South Dakota. At Yellowstone, a bear climbed on our car. Boy, did we roll up those windows fast! It was August, and we'd just been through scorching heat in the Southwest, but in the mountains of Wyoming overnight temperatures dropped below freezing. Being Canadians, we're used to cold weather. It's not so bad when you're in a heated home in Montreal; in a tent, brrrr! After visiting Mount Rushmore, we pressed on, through Madison, Wisconsin, then up into Ontario, Canada, finally ending our honeymoon back home in Montreal.

CHAPTER 4
Becoming a Doctor

The next year in Montreal was something of a transitional time for Gloria and me, as we weaved a series of endings and beginnings in and out of our lives. We each had moved out of our parents' homes for the first time, leaving behind our roles as dependent children and adjusting to our life together in our own home, as a newly married couple.

Gloria was in her teacher certification program, which was her last year of school before launching a teaching career. I was wrapping up my last year of med school, hoping to graduate successfully before starting a couple of years of rotating internship and residency.

At school, I found myself tying together the threads of my medical education, gaining a greater knowledge of the structure and functions of the human body. I developed a way of systematically thinking about the patients I was evaluating and treating in my clinical training. This involved taking a thorough history, performing a complete physical exam, and then assessing the signs and symptoms to determine what might be wrong (called a differential diagnosis) and what treatments might work for each possible diagnosis. I often found the learning painstaking and the process of acquiring medical data profound and endless. But I didn't see that as a bad thing. Gradually, I was learning the language of medicine—a language that provides the tools for the art and skill of medical reasoning. And I came to see how essential medical reasoning is, since new knowledge pours in constantly in a never-ending stream. The new information must be incorporated into a doctor's existing knowledge base with flexibility.

As all these pieces of the puzzle fell into place, I found a deeper connection to my identity and practice as a doctor. The year wore on, graduation came closer, and I grew more comfortable in my skin—my doctor's skin. I felt ready to finish the training, take my oral exams and national boards, and hopefully graduate and start my career.

I didn't, however, intend to go to my own graduation. Gloria and I were planning a trip to Europe in June. We wound up changing plans because I was asked by a department chair not to skip graduation. Turns out I'd won several significant awards, and the chairman thought I should accept them in person. I'm glad I did.

The most notable honor was the Holmes gold medal, which I earned for being top in my class, much to my surprise. I was humbled and also gratified. My commitment and hard work had paid off. I won two other prizes as well and tied for a third with Arnold Aberman, with whom I'd become friends during med school. (Arnie remains a dear friend to this day, and he contributed material for this book.) Earlier in the year, I'd won one of eight cash prizes in a contest for medical students in Canada and the US. I'd written a paper on what was then a promising new drug, allopurinol, which was being tested in the treatment of gout.

The recognition and the presence of friends and family made cancelling the European trip worthwhile. We substituted a shorter trip to Mexico. At the Mexico City airport, we met a Mexican family who invited us to their home and showed warm hospitality. From the capital, we drove to the smaller, more remote towns of Taxco and Cuernavaca. Next, we visited Acapulco and the renowned El Mirador Hotel, where we dined outdoors while watching a performance of the famous cliff divers. As souvenirs of our trip, we brought home bad sunburns from a jungle canoe ride—and a lesson about wearing sunscreen.

INTENSITY OF RESIDENCY

We were back in Montreal by the end of June 1967, and I quickly began the first rotation of my internship in what would be two years of hospital internships and residency. I was stationed for the first year at RVH, one of McGill's teaching hospitals. My father was the chief pharmacist there, and sometimes we'd commute together.

Rotating internships aren't done anymore. Interns go straight to their specialties instead. But back then, my internship consisted of three-month rotations in each of four hospital departments: pediatrics, obstetrics and gynecology, surgery, and medicine.

Surgery was my least favorite. In the operating room it was the intern's very strenuous job to hold the retractors, the tool used to hold open the wound or incision during surgery. The surgeon would put his hand on the intern's and say, "Pull harder" as he crushed their fingers until they ached. The intern also had to snip off excess sutures, something I found frustrating because I always seemed to cut them too long or too short. Overall, I wasn't well-suited for operating room work. On my rotation there, however, I eventually figured out I could avoid it by volunteering for the job of changing patient wound dressings.

Of all the rotations, I preferred my time in medicine, though it could be extremely challenging. The patients were often quite sick and their cases difficult to manage. As with many new doctors, I took it hard when any patients died on my watch. I still remember taking over the case of a comatose man with tuberculosis meningitis who did not make it and that of a young man with kidney disease who succumbed after a staph infection in his legs, swollen with fluid accumulation of edema, led to sepsis (blood poisoning) despite ample IV antibiotic therapy.

As nearly any doctor who's been through it will tell you, internships are demanding, stressful, and intensive. We work long hours on varying schedules. I was on the night shift every other day and worked every other weekend. A solid night's sleep becomes a distant memory for the typical intern, and I was no different. On-call weekends were especially grueling. That's when interns had to remain on-site at the hospital to respond quickly to patient needs and urgent situations when the attending physician was off duty and only on call.

A standard on-call weekend was flanked by regular workdays and remaining on call at the hospital through Monday morning. Then Monday would be another on-duty workday. If we were lucky, we might be able to grab a couple of hours sleep in one stretch, but it was a one-eye-open kind of sleep, since we never knew when our beeper would sound and we'd need to rush to help a patient in crisis.

Back in those days there were intern residences, sort of like dormitories, with bunk beds and small kitchens where we could, theoretically, scramble up some eggs, slide off our shoes, and drop into a bed to doze until our beeper buzzed. I say theoretically because in practice the residences could be wild places where young interns found questionable ways of burning off their stress. Being married and—as Gloria says—a goody-two-shoes, I tried to close my eyes to the hanky-panky when I closed my eyes to sleep. I couldn't shut it all out, though, and I wondered what the patients and their families would think if they knew the antics their doctors were up to behind the scenes.

On an ER rotation, we were on a four-day cycle that culminated in a twenty-hour shift, followed by twenty-four hours off duty. Sometimes I'd be too wired and wound up after a rotation to sleep. In the winter, I sometimes had my father bring my skis when he came to work. After my shift, I'd drive up to the Laurentian Mountains for a day of skiing. Sounds crazy, but it was invigorating and restorative. Leaving my stress behind on the mountainside, I'd return home and crash into bed, moribund. Then I'd wake up the next morning and head back to the hospital for my next shift.

As part of the ER rotation, interns rode along in ambulances. This is no longer done. It's not an efficient use of a doctor's time and skills, and today's emergency medical technicians are highly trained in providing the needed care. But in those days, the intern was the only qualified provider in the ambulance.

My ambulance shifts were intense, unpredictable, and sometimes scary. The hospital had one driver I remember well. His nickname was Sharky, and he always had the smell of liquor on his breath. Whether he was drunk, I don't know. Clearly, someone like Sharky would never, ever be allowed to drive an ambulance these days. Nevertheless, when the hospital would get an ambulance call for a heart attack or car crash, Sharky would be at the wheel. Since my rotation was in winter, I remember sitting white-knuckled and clench-jawed as Sharky would zoom down Montreal's snowy, icy streets, siren blaring. Thank heavens we never crashed! It was hard enough working on an ambulance without having to worry about a boozy driver.

On one gruesome call, I found a woman sitting on her toilet, where it appeared she had just delivered a baby right into the bowl. It was a nightmare; the infant was deceased. Another time, we went to a home where a woman was having abdominal pain. I noticed her belly was kind of large, but, based on her description of the pain, I thought she might be bloated and swollen from some kind of digestive tract problem. When I did a rectal exam, my finger felt something hard through the rectal wall. Imagine my shock to realize it was a baby's head. Her pains were labor pains! We rushed her back to the hospital and into the delivery room where she could safely give birth. Apparently, she was a country girl who had recently moved to the city. She didn't know she was in labor because she didn't even have a clue that she was pregnant.

In the 1994 movie *Forrest Gump*, the title character's mother (played by Sally Field) is on her deathbed when she says, "Life is a box of chocolates, Forrest. You never know what you're gonna get."[2] Such was life on ambulance calls. Sometimes you got a flavor you disliked. Other times, the chocolate was full of nuts.

BLOOD, SWEAT, AND . . . FECES?

In late-1960s Montreal, interns were paid $4,000 a year. Yes, the dollar went a whole lot further than now. But think of the volume of hours we clocked, on duty and on call. We were easily putting in two to three times the work of an average full-time job. Add to that the wide variety of tasks we were required to perform, whether or not they related to what would eventually be our practice of medicine. Sometimes, when we were dragging at the heels from exhaustion or

---

[2] *Forrest Gump*, directed by Robert Zemeckis (1994, Los Angeles, CA: Paramount Pictures, 2001), DVD.

our hands were being painfully squeezed by arrogant surgeons, interns and residents felt very much like cheap, exploited labor.

The hospital provided us with uniforms consisting of white shirts and white pants. In the mornings, those of us on the ward team of white-clad doctors toured the floor, rolling a cart used for drawing blood. This was before the contemporary era, when blood is drawn by certified, specialized technicians. Back then, we interns did the work. Drawing blood safely and painlessly is a skill that takes some learning, and here we were, practicing on our patients' arms. Honestly, I often felt bad for the patients as we approached them holding a large, 50-milliliter glass syringe, especially since we were still gaining the skills to draw blood competently.

We multi-purpose interns were also tasked with a job that was downright primitive by today's standards: We ran urinalyses and testing stool for occult (hidden) blood. Nowadays this is always, unfailingly, done in a laboratory under safe and sterile conditions. But in our medical Stone Age of the 1960s, we used a small side room right on the wards. I'm probably understating it when I say this was a disgusting, unsanitary place with the foul stench of human waste we tried unsuccessfully to ignore.

I was working in this wretched excuse for a lab one day, wearing my tidy, white uniform. In a moment of clumsiness, I spilled a container of feces on myself. Ugh, putrid! I rapidly fled the room to find a shower and a fresh uniform, determined to use more caution in the future to avoid such a mishap, even if that meant going slower on the job. The good news for patients and doctors today is that these smelly, germy side rooms have been abolished. As have many of the extraneous duties heaped onto interns and residents, who are now able to focus more on the care and treatment of sick people.

I once had a patient with just one arm. He had what we call a GI bleed (bleeding from the gastrointestinal tract). He was vomiting blood and had other symptoms indicating he was in danger and needed urgent attention. I tried to insert an intravenous line so that we could quickly get medicine into his system. As with drawing blood, intravenous insertion takes a great deal of know-how and experience. Typically, when there's difficulty placing it in one arm, you try the other. That wasn't possible here. The man was getting sicker. This was physically hard on him and nerve-wracking for me. Finally, I called in a senior resident who was able to get the job done.

These kinds of experiences typified the unpredictable, arduous, and ever-changing world of hospital interns and residents. But despite the seeming craziness of it all, most doctors were passionate, competent, and devoted to their work.

It was shortly into my second year of this wild, woolly, and sleep-deprived hospital training that I had my first episode with the scintillating scotoma while sitting alone in Lenny Diamond's car. Now that you have a contextual picture of who I was and what my life was like before my illness and hospitalization, we'll get back to the surprising and mysterious events that unfolded for me in 1968 and 1969.

CHAPTER 5
My Health Races Downhill

Let's check back in with that young man sitting forlorn and frightened in the ER, waiting for the resident neurologist to do an exam. It was a Friday evening, November 29, 1968. A little earlier, Dr. Gault had found me in the parking lot outside his office, disoriented and waving my finger in front of my face. I had just had my second incident of a flashing blue light appearing in front of my eyes, temporarily blinding me on the left side. The medical records I reviewed decades later said that along with the flashing light, I reported nausea, confusion, and a worsening headache.

Dr. Gault had led me back into his office, where we'd been working together shortly before, and he looked me over. Although the blue light had disappeared and my vision would soon be restored, he drove me to the ER at RVH. For my part, I was already writing my epitaph. I'd persuaded myself the symptoms pointed to a brain tumor that would probably kill me and, if not, shatter my career prospects. In a matter of minutes, a simple flash of light had derailed my straight-ahead, on-track life and promising future. Well, at least that was the doomsday tale I created in my head.

Having done one of my three-month intern rotations at the RVH ER, I was quite familiar with the place. But it's a whole other kettle of fish when you're there as a worried patient.

With limited success, I tried to maintain my professional demeanor as I waited for the neurology resident to examine me. When Gloria and my parents arrived, I had a support team, though I could see they were as anxious and unsettled as I was by this unexpected turn of events. In my personal account written back then, I noted that my mother showed her concern by chattering almost nonstop, while my father kept patting me on the head.

After I saw the neurologist, the ER team decided to send me home. My symptoms had gone, and they couldn't pinpoint anything immediately wrong with me. They must have taken my condition seriously, though, because they set me up with an appointment the very next day, Saturday, with Dr. Francis McNaughton, the chief of neurology at MNH.

From the ER, the four of us headed home for what was to be a night of great anxiety for me. I was still caught in the doomsday scenario I'd constructed, convinced I had a malignant brain tumor. Not just any brain tumor, mind you, but the most aggressive, deadly, and hard-to-treat brain cancer—glioblastoma. And while I was in the business of self-diagnosing, I kept going and issued a prognosis: the glioblastoma would kill me within a year.

DIFFERENTIAL DIAGNOSIS: A LESSON NOT LEARNED

It's funny. In hindsight, I can see the irony of my predicament. I'm not saying this in self-deprecation; I have compassion for the panic I was feeling. Rather, I'm sharing my belatedly learned lesson because it may prove helpful to people confronted with a medical crisis that's replete with unknowns.

Less than a year and a half before this incident, I had graduated first in my class from McGill University Medical School. With immense and sometimes painstaking effort,

I gradually grew fluent in the language of medicine. At its most basic level, this language describes, measures, tests, and treats the structure and functions of the body and its interactions with its habitat—that is, the objects, substances, and organisms that humans encounter every minute of every day. This language provides the tools for medical reasoning, which is an essential skill because a doctor draws from a well of knowledge that's complex, ever-expanding, and ever-changing.

I learned a way of systematically thinking about the sick patients I cared for during my two clinical years of med school. This was crucial to becoming a competent doctor who is skilled in the foundational practice known as differential diagnosis. You see, people go to doctors with symptoms, not diseases. A patient shows up in the office and cries, "Doc, I'm peeing blood!" Then it's a detective job to figure out what's causing the symptom in order to plot out the best therapy.

The differential diagnostic process can sometimes be very straightforward, say, for example, when a patient comes into the ER with a gash in their hand from a bagel-slicing mishap. But it's often more complicated and involves several components: conducting a physical exam, taking the patient's medical history, and ordering lab work, imaging, or other studies. Doctors apply their medical knowledge and experience, plus they must know how to find more information and assistance if needed. Integrating all these components can be like piecing together a multi-dimensional jigsaw puzzle, working without a picture of the result.

So when that patient thinks they have blood in their urine, the doctor takes a thorough history and does a physical exam. The doctor considers all possible diseases and conditions that may cause blood in the urine and matches that knowledge with findings from the history and exam. This narrows down the options and determines which kinds of tests and images are best to elicit an answer. Possible causes are numerous. Is it bladder cancer? Kidney stones? Urinary infection? Medication? Maybe the patient's Ukrainian grandma made them a delicious pot of borscht the night before. (Eating beets can color the urine red.)

This comprehensive process requires an open mind, with the understanding that there's always more to learn. Doctors have to be flexible and adaptable to new information as it becomes available. We saw this with the COVID-19 pandemic in so many ways, such as how the coronavirus spread between people. At first, we thought it spread on surfaces. Turns out it was primarily spread through the air. Medical knowledge is never static, nor is the course of human health.

Why am I telling you all this about differential diagnosis? For one thing, it's important for people facing tough medical situations to know their health providers are using an organized, systematic approach to figuring out what's wrong. They work methodically with a vast array of information to come to a sound and well-reasoned conclusion, or at least a list of strong finalists for the source of the illness.

In November of 1968, I was a practitioner who had helped many patients by systematically applying my knowledge, medical reasoning, and diagnostic skills to come to logical plans of action about the likely causes of the illnesses and optimal treatments. And when I suddenly came down with disturbing and unusual symptoms of my own, did I adopt the same deliberative approach to my own diagnosis? Nope! Did I wait until the elements of differential diagnosis were performed and all the data was collected before forming an opinion? No again. Therein lies the irony.

This outcome exemplifies why doctors should never care for their health problems by self-diagnosing and treating.

They should always have another doctor manage their illness. Emotions such as dread, panic, and anger cloud the mind, overpowering the rational, cognitive processes associated with the parts of the brain responsible for coherent thinking and reasoning. Instead of reminding myself to wait until all the facts were in, I latched onto a single med-school memory of a doctor with similar symptoms caused by a brain tumor. I snatched up that idea like a pickpocket grabs a wallet, then let my mind leap to the most tragic outcomes.

While it was true that I might have had a brain tumor, jumping to that conclusion was premature. I didn't need my medical skills, I needed emotional ones—patience, calmness, and a willingness to keep my mind open to the various possibilities that would present themselves once all the facts were gathered. Despite my medical expertise, in that moment of fear I didn't have an advantage over someone who doesn't know the difference between a coronary artery and a tunnel from Logan Airport to Boston.

Some people call this mental state "don't-know mind." Now, that doesn't refer to ignorance. It's kind of a mental practice of remembering that your thoughts and opinions are formed from the best knowledge available at present and holding an intellectual door open to new data that may change your options. It's not easy, but anyone can prepare to respond to a crisis in this way. Then, when something happens—and it inevitably will—they'll be more prepared to act calmly, make better decisions, and maybe help bring about a better outcome.

On the eve of World War II in the summer of 1939, the British government anticipated that major cities in the country were going to be subject to a blitz—a massive aerial bombardment by the Germans. Looking to boost morale and prevent panic in the event of such an onslaught, the Ministry of Information designed a poster bearing the phrase "Keep Calm and Carry On" under a drawing of a crown. The government printed up more than two million of these bright red-and-white posters, and then never circulated them.

The famous English "stiff upper lip" seemed to get most citizens through the immense hardships of the war without benefit of the poster. It was forgotten for decades until 2000, when the owner of a used bookstore found an original poster in a box of old books and displayed it in his shop. The phrase resonated with customers, who began buying reprints of the posters. Around 2008, when the Great Recession hit, the slogan exploded into a widely popular commercial meme, with the graphic appearing on mugs, T-shirts, greeting cards, tattoos—you name it.

No doctor will write you a prescription to "Keep Calm and Carry On." Luckily, it's safe to use without one. Store it in a figurative back pocket of your mind or create your own comparable mantra. When you find yourself suddenly consumed by fear in the face of a crisis, those few simple words might be enough to jolt you awake and keep you from falling down the rabbit hole of panic and perceived catastrophe. You'll still have to go through all the tests, exams, procedures, etcetera, but you'll be able to do it with a clearer mind that will enable better decision-making.

HURRAY, I'VE GOT MIGRAINES!

On the Saturday after my ER visit, I went for a follow-up appointment with Dr. McNaughton. He was also a highly respected professor at McGill and had been one of my teachers there. He was renowned for his scientific work on the anatomical basis for understanding and treating headaches, as well as for the diagnosis and treatment of epilepsy.

Dr. McNaughton was a superb neurologist who was smart and talented. He had a rare combination of all the attributes you want in a doctor: skill, broad expertise, gentleness, compassion, and a willingness to take the time needed to provide the highest quality care to his patients. He was a fabulous clinical professor and a wonderful human being, with a soft-spoken, friendly manner that inspired trust. His expertise was fortuitous, given the medical ordeal I was soon to endure. He took care of me throughout my hospitalizations at MNH and continued to participate in my care after I was transferred to a psychiatric hospital.

In his office, Dr. McNaughton evaluated me thoroughly and saw that my neurological findings were all normal. He considered the headaches I'd been having and the visual disturbance of the flashing blue light, which was accompanied by the loss of sight on the same side of the visual field of both my eyes. This occurrence is known as *homonymous hemianopsia*. In my case, it was transient. Dr. McNaughton came to the opinion that the flashing blue light and my transient loss of vision were due to an aura associated with migraine headaches. An aura is a sensory or perceptual disturbance. Specifically, I had a visual aura, which actually has nothing to do with eyesight but is caused by some communications problems in the brain. An aura usually acts as a kind of warning that a migraine attack is beginning or about to begin.

Things would change again in a couple of days when I would develop new symptoms, but for the moment I breathed an enormous sigh of relief. While most people wouldn't think of a migraine diagnosis as a cause for celebration, I was elated. Remember that I'd convinced myself I had a terminal brain tumor and only a matter of months to live. Now I sat listening to a doctor I respected who was saying I had migraines—an unpleasant, but eminently manageable condition. I felt like a death row prisoner who'd been granted clemency and freed from prison!

SEIZED

My early diagnosis wasn't much of a reprieve, lasting only a couple of days. Dr. McNaughton came to his differential diagnosis based on a thorough review of the evidence that was available to him at the time. When he diagnosed me as having a migraine with aura, he was fully aware that an aura can also occur with an epileptic seizure. After all, he was an expert in both areas. Since I had a headache with the aura and had never experienced a seizure, Dr. McNaughton concluded I had migraines.

During that period, I was assigned to a rotation at the Royal Edward Laurentian Chest Hospital in Montreal, where many of the patients had lung cancer or tuberculosis. On Monday morning, two days after seeing Dr. McNaughton, I returned to work as scheduled. It was December 2, 1968.

I was at the nurses' station in the evening when the flashing blue light appeared again. By chance, Dr. Arnie Aberman phoned just then. Arnie and I attended med school together and had been friends since we first met in 1960. When he called that night, he was on his shift in rotation at a different hospital. Arnie knew of my migraine diagnosis two days before. When I got on the phone, I said, "Arnie, I am having my migraine." That's the last thing I remember. As part of my research some fifty years later, I interviewed Arnie. He recalls that the phone seemed to go dead at that point.

"I was speaking with you, Irving, and all of a sudden, it falls dead. I didn't know what was going on. I was saying, 'Irving, Irving' and a nurse picked up the phone and told me you just had a seizure."

I guess being in a hospital and surrounded by medical professionals is a good place to have this happen. In my hospital admission report, there was a remarkably detailed account of my seizure that was presumably provided by the nurse and/or other clinical staff on duty. Dr. J. Armstrong, a neurology resident at MNH, wrote in the admitting report, *Tonight, he experienced yet a third episode of his visual disturbance, together with an exacerbation of his headache. He again was nauseated, and while talking on the telephone to one of his friends, he suddenly had a generalized tonic-clonic convulsion. This began with a twitching on the left corner of his face, followed by collapse, and flexion of the left arm.* Dr. Armstrong said that fifteen minutes later, I was "drowsy, but oriented, and had amnesia for the event." I could only remember up to the point that my headache got worse and I felt nauseated.

To cover some basics, a seizure is a sudden burst of electrical activity in the brain that is uncontrolled and causes symptoms elsewhere in the brain and body. A generalized seizure happens when the abnormal electrical signals occur in both hemispheres of the brain at the same time. A tonic-clonic seizure, once known as a grand mal seizure, typically comes in two stages, starting with the tonic part when the muscles stiffen and the person loses consciousness and collapses. They may groan, gurgle, or cry out. The second, clonic stage is what most people probably envision when they think of seizures, with strong contractions and jerking of the muscles in the arms, legs, and face. The whole thing lasts just a few minutes, although the patient may not regain consciousness for a little while longer. Sleepiness, confusion, and mood alternations may occur in the wake of the seizure, and the headache may persist.

I have a faint memory of waking up in a hospital bed feeling groggy and confused. I remember reaching into my trousers to determine whether I had wet myself, since it's known that urinary incontinence often occurs during a seizure; I wasn't wet. Staff raced me by ambulance from the chest hospital to MNH, where they specialize in neurological issues such as mine. I was admitted to MNH and remained there for eleven days, under the supervision of Dr. McNaughton.

You may be wondering whether Dr. McNaughton made an error when he diagnosed the flashing blue light as a migraine with aura. No, he made the right call based on his assessment of the available evidence. This is when the physician's attribute of flexibility comes into play. Two days later, the set of facts was modified by my first seizure. It was now clear that the visual disturbance was the aura for a seizure. We had a new ball game.

MY FIRST HOSPITALIZATION

In a sense, the ambulance didn't just transport me from one hospital to another; it brought me to a new world. I was no longer a doctor with the power and authority to help people in need of care. Now I was on the other end of the stethoscope—sick, vulnerable, helpless, and uncertain what was wrong with me or what lay in store.

Day or night, with little to no warning, I was subject to being scanned, scrutinized, and sedated; poked, prodded, and punctured. I lost my privacy, with all my body parts and functions laid bare, open to examination and discussion by strangers. Don't get me wrong. I'm deeply grateful for the superb, high-quality care I received. But perhaps it was a blessing that I remembered so little of that three-month period.

My first admission to Montreal Neurological Hospital (MNH) lasted from December 2–13, 1968. On December 7, Gloria and my brother Allan came in to celebrate my twenty-fifth birthday with me. I recall that first hospitalization about as well as the passing of more than fifty years allows. My memory has been refreshed a little by the personal narrative I wrote during my illness, and I think most of my other two hospital stints would be blank pages had I not been able to acquire my complete medical records from the hospitals. Those encompassed the period during which I developed serious psychiatric illness. The documents are detailed and thorough, and they've helped me piece together a chronicle of my extraordinary medical journey.

Dr. Armstrong wrote the admitting report, but the discharge summary has Dr. McNaughton's name on it, so I'll consider him the author. For organizational reasons, I'm going to focus here on the clinical findings, and later we'll look more at the personal aspects and how this impacted me. The big-picture purposes of my hospital care were threefold: 1) to treat and alleviate my symptoms, 2) to prevent any more seizures, and 3) to find the cause of my illness.

I had a second seizure sometime later that night or early the next morning. It happened in Dr. Armstrong's presence, right after he'd examined me upon admission to MNH. He wrote that it started with my having a *peculiar abdominal sensation, with some nausea, exacerbation of his headache. This was accompanied by a blue flashing light again in the left upper quadrant of the visual field, and prior to the onset of his seizure, he had a left homonymous hemianopsia.*

Dr. Armstrong then wrote that the seizure began with twitching of my facial muscles and movement of my head to the left. The convulsion then became generalized, with stiffening and some jerking of my left arm: *This jerking then ceased, and the whole body became rigid, stiff, and cyanosed. The patient took on a deadly purple colour and was almost unrecognizable.* Continuing, he noted that the convulsion lasted less than two minutes, followed by a period of stupor: *Gradually patient regained consciousness, although he continued to be somewhat drowsy for 15 or 20 minutes. He answered questions inappropriately as to time. Eventually he recognized me and could carry on a sensible conversation.* I was briefly dizzy, and had a bad headache, nausea, and sleepiness.

Dr. Armstrong's report then goes on to give full details of my examination and history. He concludes that I had *focal cerebral seizures, originating in the right cerebral hemisphere, probably in parietal-occipital region, and undetermined etiology.* In his discharge summary, Dr. McNaughton also described me as having focal cerebral seizures. Unlike generalized seizures that start in both hemispheres of the brain, focal seizures begin in only one hemisphere.

So, if I had two generalized tonic-clonic seizures, then why do my reports say focal seizures? It's because careful observations by witnesses revealed that the initial manifestations were symptoms of focal seizures, not generalized. The location where a focal seizure starts predicts what the symptoms will be. Seizures begin with abnormal electrical impulses. A focal seizure sends out signals that may trigger other neurons (brain cells) to send out impulses of their own. It can have a sort of cascading effect that leads to a full-blown tonic-clonic seizure.

To put it another way, the doctors investigating a seizure want to know where in the brain it originated because that brings them closer to identifying the cause. In my case, both neurologists realized that the stronger tonic-clonic seizures had followed a milder focal seizure. When Dr. Armstrong wrote that my seizures were of undetermined etiology, that simply means "cause unknown." They would need to collect and analyze more data to help them solve the puzzle, or at least make some educated guesses about the cause. And they'd be collecting that data from me in a series of sampling and imaging procedures that would make my life rather unpleasant in the coming days.

Dr. Armstrong noted that my seizures originated in the right hemisphere, most likely in the parietal-occipital region. Located in the very back of the head, the occipital lobes—one in each brain hemisphere—are mainly responsible for the ability to understand what the eyes are seeing. The aura and seizure incidents I experienced impacted my sight and visual fields, which implicated the occipital lobe. He knew it was the right hemisphere because I'd had symptoms that affected the left side, including the transient loss of vision and the left-side facial twitching that occurred at the beginning of my focal seizures. There's a sort of crisscrossing effect, when the right side of the brain controls actions on the left side of the vision and face. The human brain is a truly remarkable thing!

Sight is actually a long series of steps that occur in far less time than the blink of an eye. When you look at an object, the light reflected from it enters your eyes and is projected onto the retina upside down and two-dimensional. Much the way a computer converts information to code, the retinal cells change the light into electrical signals that move along through the optic nerve and into the brain. The brain processes the various features, such as color, and then sort of reassembles the electrical impulses back into an image, one that's right side up and three-dimensional. Only then can you understand what you're seeing.

Other than the fact that I'd just had two powerful seizures, Dr. Armstrong's evaluation of my condition upon admission to MNH was remarkably unremarkable. He noted that I'd had a cold and cough for a few weeks. I told him that over the prior two weeks, I felt like I'd lost a bit of my intellectual sharpness, something that was evident in my chess game and an increased tendency to misplace things. Through my work at the chest hospital, I had frequent exposure to tuberculosis, an infectious disease that occasionally causes brain infections. But I'd been vaccinated about five years earlier and had recently done a test that was negative. Thus, tuberculosis was ruled out as a cause of my illness.

Dr. Armstrong also added in his notes, *The patient has been bothered most of his adult life by a rather severe case of facial acne, and for the last couple of months has been treating himself with tetracycline, at a dose averaging 500 mg. a day.* Tetracycline is an antibiotic that's still sometimes used to treat bad acne. Dr. Armstrong apparently kept up on his pharmacology, because he mentioned a study in the medical literature that *incriminated this substance as a cause of increased intracranial pressure.* Since 1968, further studies have confirmed that this effect sometimes occurs. To help explain, cerebrospinal fluid (CSF) is a clear liquid that surrounds the brain and spinal cord (the central nervous system). When the volume of CSF increases inside the skull, it puts pressure on the brain. Could a rise in intracranial pressure cause seizures? There's a chance, which is why Dr. Armstrong mentioned it. But he thought the possibility was remote: *As an etiology of this patient's seizures, it is probably unlikely.* Dr. McNaughton must have agreed, since he didn't even mention tetracycline in his discharge report.

In the search for clues to the cause of my seizures, the doctors ran plenty of tests, scans, and studies on me. They tested my blood and urine, checked my biochemistry and immunochemistry, and ran a long and nasty glucose tolerance test to check my blood sugar. They checked for lymphocytes in my CSF and did find an elevated level. Lymphocytes are a type of white blood cell, and an elevation often indicates inflammation of the brain. Several things may cause brain inflammation, including infection.

In addition, I underwent a pneumoencephalogram, a test to look for brain tumors or brain scarring that could cause seizures. This test is no longer used today, having been supplanted by far better imaging technology, such as magnetic resonance imaging (better known as MRI) and computed tomography (better known as CT or CAT scan). Good riddance! A pneumoencephalogram involved inserting a needle into the spine to drain the CSF from around the brain and then replacing the fluid with injected air. Next they'd take an image of the brain using X-ray technology with the air to contrast the outline of the brain. This offered a better picture of the brain, especially to look for lesions or damaged tissue. It was a painful and uncomfortable process because it required puncturing the lumbar (lower) spine to drain the CSF and inject air. A pneumoencephalogram was bad enough under the best of circumstances. Mine was made even worse by a thoughtless nurse who taunted me. She bragged about her own experience with the procedure and made sure to tell me it was the doctor's first time performing it. They also had no proper sedative available to make it easier for me.

The pneumoencephalogram X-rays didn't produce any significant finds, but the procedure was important since no brain tumor or brain scarring were detected. I also had a transbrachial angiogram to check my carotid artery as well as a vertebral angiogram. Both procedures require needle punctures and catheter insertion, and both cause significant discomfort. Findings from both were deemed normal.

I also endured two electroencephalograms (better known as EEGs), during which they induced me to hyperventilate, something that enhances the image results when looking for abnormalities from seizures or epilepsy. These EEGs did show some slight abnormalities, but nothing that offered any clear answers. My brain scan was normal.

As for medications, they put me on Dilantin, an anti-seizure medication that can prevent both tonic-clonic and focal seizures. It has numerous side effects, a few of which can be serious. They also gave me phenobarbital (sometimes called phenobarb), a central nervous system depressant that's an effective anti-seizure drug but is also addictive and prone to abuse due to its strongly sedating effects. Both drugs were absolutely necessary for me to take to prevent seizures, and they helped. But the side effects of phenobarbital may be part of the reason I remember almost nothing about my hospitalization for psychiatric problems. And they may also account for some of the troubles I had that you'll read about in the next chapter.

In his discharge summary, Dr. McNaughton recommended that I continue with Dilantin and phenobarb after I went home. He wanted me to return for another EEG in a month's time. He concluded his discharge summary on December 13th with a diagnosis that said, "Viral encephalitis suspected." Encephalitis is an inflammation of the brain. Among the many things that can cause it is a virus.

Dr. McNaughton's diagnosis meant the doctors were inching closer to finding the cause of my condition. He wrote, *the various investigations, mainly the increase in CSF cells, pointed towards inflammatory process, and it was felt this was probably a viral encephalitis, although no virus was isolated.* That wasn't exactly the definitive kind of answer I was hoping for as I prepared to resume my normal activities. The solution remained elusive, as it does for many individuals who go through health crises.

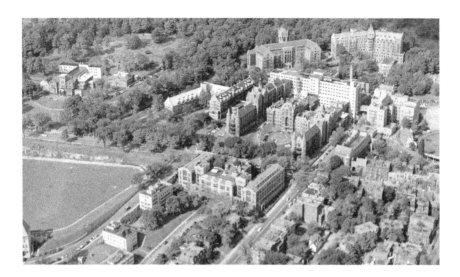

In the center is an Aerial view of the Royal Victoria Hospital (RVH). To the right of RVH across a small street is the Montreal Neurological Institute and Hospital. To the far left is the Allan Memorial Institute. From McGill University Archives Pro23742, 1954.

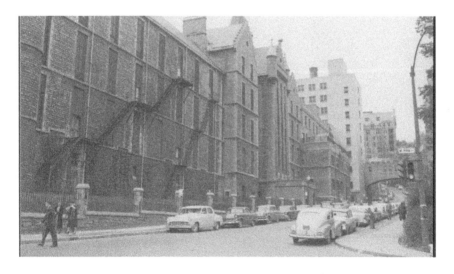

The surgical ward and outpatient department of the Royal Victoria Hospital as viewed from the corner of Pine Avenue and University Avenue. The elevated crosswalk on the right connects to Montreal Neurological Hospital. The view looked much the same in 2022 although the cars are different. From McGill University Archives PRO23732, 1954. This same picture was used for the book cover.

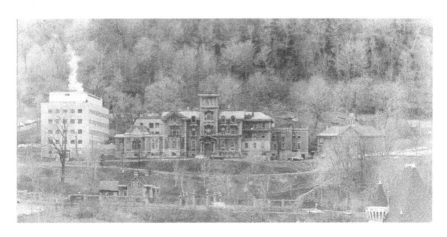

The exterior of the Allan Memorial Institute in 1970.
From McGill University Archives PRO45091.

CHAPTER 6

A Glimmer of Hope Dimmed by New Obstacles

By today's standards, an eleven-day hospital stay is something of a marathon, particularly for a twenty-five-year-old who was in robust, good health just weeks earlier. Longer stays weren't all that unusual in 1968, the days before insurance coverage limits and payment caps shrank the average length of a hospital stay to the bare minimum. Still, my hospitalization was a long haul, a physical and emotional ordeal, and a disruptive experience for my family and me.

It felt as if an earthquake had struck. And while the temblor didn't knock down the house, we didn't know whether it had damaged the foundation enough to make the building unstable. My medical team had made progress on a diagnosis by ruling out unviable options, yet much remained shrouded in darkness. Viral encephalitis moved front and center as the lineup of "usual suspects" was whittled down. The diagnosis was qualified as "suspected" viral encephalitis. As to what actual virus might have infected my brain and where I caught it, those were question marks too.

I emerged from MNH having celebrated my milestone twenty-fifth birthday in a hospital bed. My careful and thorough providers tested, assessed, and treated me down to the last minute. Instead of going home, Gloria and I went to my parents' house in the city of Côte Saint-Luc on the island of Montreal. It made sense to have more people around me, especially with Gloria leaving every day for her job teaching seventh grade. As the chief pharmacist at RVH, my father commanded a wealth of knowledge on diseases and treatments and was well-positioned to oversee my recuperation. What a blessing to have my family pull together to support me!

I have only fragmentary memories of that week after discharge. As a family, I'm sure we all felt collective relief that I'd made it through what we thought was the worst of my illness. There'd been no seizures since that first night in the hospital, an indication that I was likely responding well to medication. My worst fear—a brain tumor—was almost certainly off the table as a possibility. My condition was frightening and ambiguous, but the Grim Reaper's breath was not upon me.

Judging by our actions in the day or two after my discharge, my family and I made a slight shift towards the optimistic belief that normalcy and good health would promptly return. Yes, we were living on tenterhooks about what the future held. Yes, I was given anti-seizure medication with side effects that impaired my memory and dulled my previously sharp mind. At the same time, we chose to behave as if I were getting well. It was quite the mixed bag. For my family, it must have been a delicate balancing act to encourage a speedy return to health while keeping a wary eye out for trouble. Some ominous signs of further decline would present themselves very soon.

THE LITTLE PRINCE

In Côte Saint-Luc, I came across a copy of the beloved fable and modern classic *The Little Prince* by Antoine de

Saint-Exupéry. I'm not sure how I got it, as I'd never read it or had it read to me as a child. But there I was with this children's book in my hands, and for some reason I started reading. I found it revelatory, powerful, and profound. I told people it held the secrets to the meaning of life. Gloria described my reaction as "over-exuberant." For a time, I was totally preoccupied, even obsessed with the story and its significance.

Saint-Exupéry was born into a French aristocratic family. A competitive global aviator and accomplished writer, he became a military combat pilot early in World War II, fighting with the Free French Air Force until France fell to the Germans in 1940. He and his wife then fled to New York, where he wrote and illustrated *The Little Prince*. It was published in the US in 1943. In France, where the pro-Nazi Vichy government banned Saint-Exupéry's works, his book didn't come out until 1946, after liberation—posthumously. Longing to help his country, Saint-Exupéry rejoined the Free French Air Force in 1943. He was lost on a mission in 1944 when his plane was believed shot down by the enemy.

The story's narrator is a pilot who conveys a lesson he learned as a child: that adults are narrow-minded, unimaginative, and literally unable to see the important things in life as they truly are. Children, meanwhile, are wise because they are open-minded; willing to explore, learn, and withhold judgement; and able to see through superficial material facades. When the pilot's plane crashes in a remote desert, he meets a little prince, a magical young boy with golden curls and fantastical tales.

The prince's home is a tiny asteroid in space. He has come to Earth after leaving his home and traveling among the stars. The stories he tells the narrator of his travels are parables of flawed adult human nature. In his adventures, the prince meets a fox who expresses the moral of the story with these words: "It is only in the heart that one can see rightly; what is essential is invisible to the eye."[3]

Is that the profound insight I felt back in 1968 and tried to convey to everyone around me? No idea. As part of my research in 2020, I reread *The Little Prince* and found it delightfully enchanting. It did not, however, evoke deep meaning or conjure any emotional or philosophical memories of my first reading. It's a bit of a comical twist that my medications, my brain's electrical misfiring, or my physical and emotional frailty may have put me in the kind of child-like, open-minded state that Saint-Exupéry described. A half century of adulthood later, is my mind perhaps a little less open and curious? Gloria characterizes me as being fixated with *The Little Prince* and hyperbolizing its meaning: "You were seeing things that you magnified as being wonderful. It was as if you had taken some psychedelic drugs." To be clear, Gloria was describing a change she observed in my mental status. The drugs I was taking at that point to prevent seizures—Dilantin and phenobarbital—wouldn't have had any effects or side effects that would fall into the category of what we think of as psychedelic. My mental condition was indeed declining, but it wasn't due to my treatments. As you'll see, there were other reasons for my increasingly erratic behavior.

YELLOW SUBMARINE

Speaking of psychedelics, the groundbreaking animated Beatles movie *Yellow Submarine* is filled with bright and psychedelic colors, visual effects, and sounds. Released in 1968, *Yellow Submarine* reinvented the animation genre in a multitude of ways, adding layers of maturity and sophistication

---

[3.] Antoine de Saint-Exupéry, *The Little Prince*, trans. Richard Howard (San Diego: Harcourt, 2000), 63.

to the themes, stories, and production, thus creating a broad appeal to adults. Previously, animated films had been largely dominated by Disney style and were made almost exclusively for children.

The film features the song of the same name, which was a smash hit when it came out two years earlier on the Beatles album *Revolver* and as a single. The song was written primarily by Paul McCartney, with a little help from his friend and bandmate John Lennon. McCartney composed a happy ditty about a happy place, intended for children, and it was produced in a way that kids would love.

Based on the simple, kid-friendly nature of the song and the cartoon style, Gloria and my brother Allan thought it would be an enjoyable, light-hearted outing for me, a day or two after my release from MNH. It seemed like a good way to ease me back into normalcy. Unfortunately, it didn't work out as anticipated. For photosensitive people, strobe lights, flashing or flickering lights, quick cuts, some types of patterns, and other visual effects can trigger seizures and other symptoms, such as nausea and vomiting.

Gloria and Allan had the best of intentions in taking me to see *Yellow Submarine*. In the theatre, they began to worry that the lights and effects might initiate a seizure in me. Thankfully, it didn't. But I do recall finding the visuals extremely uncomfortable. Whether that discomfort included nausea or any other symptoms, I don't remember. I believe we may have left before the film ended. These incidents pointed to deteriorating mental processes and early signs of psychosis. (Psychosis is characterized by a loss of contact with reality.)

My brother Allan was still in medical school at McGill at the time. He went on to become a preeminent, world-renowned interventional neuroradiologist, researcher, and professor, with many publications and awards to his name.

As part of my effort to reconstruct the events of my illness, I interviewed him in 2020 and asked about the trip to see *Yellow Submarine*.

"It was innovative," he said. "It had all the psychedelic stuff. It was disturbing stuff and we realized when we were there that this wasn't right for you because you were already in a worried state. Then a few days later, you evolved into psychosis. So I don't know if the film contributed to the developing psychosis, but I felt guilty about taking you there."

Looking back, I think it's likely that guilt was unwarranted, and we can let both Allan and *Yellow Submarine* off the hook.

RETURN TO WORK: THE CRAZIEST DAY OF MY LIFE

Let's quickly recap the timeline up to this point. On an unspecified date in November of 1968, I had a brief flashing-light episode that was quickly forgotten. On November 29 of the same year, I had a similar occurrence, this time with a bad headache, temporary loss of left-side vision, confusion, and other symptoms. Those symptoms sent me to the ER, where everything seemed normal, so I went home.

In a follow-up appointment the next day, a neurologist diagnosed the flashing light as an aura for a migraine. Two days later, I experienced the aura and then collapsed with a generalized seizure while talking on the phone at work. That effectively erased the migraine diagnosis and replaced it with an aura for seizures. I was rushed by ambulance to MNH, where I had another seizure shortly after admission. I stayed at MNH for eleven days and was discharged on Friday, December 13, with a best-guess diagnosis of possible viral encephalitis and prescriptions for two strong anti-seizure drugs.

After discharge, my wife and I went to stay at my parents' house. Over that weekend, I became fixated with the revelations I discovered in *The Little Prince*. At the movies, the visual effects in *Yellow Submarine* caused me great discomfort. My mental status was in decline, but I didn't realize it—or maybe I did but thought I could conquer the situation through sheer strength of will. I told myself that my release from the hospital and the lack of further seizures meant I was well. In a personal observation, sort of a journal entry that I wrote at the time, I referred to having "feelings of definitive doom in the near future."

My identity revolved around being a good, hard-working doctor, and I had a strong desire to return to my duties and get back to normal. Acting against medical advice, I returned to work at the Royal Laurentian Chest Hospital on Monday, December 16—less than three days after my hospital release. It was a harrowing experience for me. While my memories of so much of this period are sparse, I have a reliable eyewitness account in my own detailed reporting of the day's events, some of which I'll be quoting in this recounting.

"My wife told me that my first day at work would be the worst day of my life. I accepted her opinion with an amused tolerance. Little did I know that her words would prove to be totally and completely true."

I headed off to work in the morning feeling calm and collected, having tamped down my "emotional problem" of that overpowering feeling of impending doom the day before. Walking into the hospital brought my first hint of trouble to come. "I suddenly realized that the belt for my uniform trousers was still at home on the door." I was understandably averse to the idea of my pants dropping 'round my ankles as I examined a patient or spoke with colleagues, so I found a smaller pair that was tight enough to stay up without a belt. Whew, one problem solved.

Things went smoothly after that, until after lunch when I was in a doctors' conference titled "Pulmonary Function" and got a call telling me I was needed on the ward to examine a young female patient who needed a doctor immediately. She was Greek and spoke only a few words of English. "What hurts?" I asked, and she pointed to the upper-left quadrant of her abdomen, where I could feel that her spleen was enlarged. I didn't think it was urgent and went back to the conference.

"But while sitting in the discussion, I had a sense of urgency." As part of the conference, I was asked a question about the significance of some lab results. "Thoughts were shut off from my mind and I just stood there like a dumb idiot and could not speak. Never in all my life did I feel so completely stupid." The moment the conference was over, I went straight back to the Greek patient's room. Her husband translated as I took a complete history.

"I could not believe it. She had all the worst symptoms. I looked at her, and she was sick, and each symptom was true. Fever, cold, spitting blood, bloody diarrhea which was nocturnal, and urinary frequency at night." Though she was the ill one, I wrote, "As the facts became revealed, I felt sicker and sicker. I couldn't believe it. My first day back at work, a nervous wreck, and I had this very ill girl on my hands, and I did not have a clue what she had." I thought maybe leukemia, but there were no other supporting indicators.

"Then I decided she needed blood tests immediately. Naturally, I missed my first venipuncture and allowed the nurse to proceed." The nurse drew the blood sample, and as I walked out of the room I noticed the patient's husband looked funny, though I quickly forgot about it. I was on the phone when I heard the nurses yelling for me. There was an emergency.

"I got off the phone and ran to the room where the patient's husband was on the floor and looked dead. He is too young for a heart attack! No pulse! Impossible! Cardiac arrest!" I called a code to bring in the resuscitation team to revive him. Then I felt his pulse again and realized my reports of his death were premature—he had only fainted. "How stupid of me, cancel it [the code]. Oops, too late! What an ass I am. I was never so embarrassed in all my life. Disbelief in what was happening struck me. There was no confidence in myself."

With the husband attended to, I turned back to his wife. "When I examined the patient just after this episode, I could hardly hear anything. I was totally uncertain of any finding that was elicited. But the abnormalities were definitely there, and I did not have a clue what they meant."

It's hard to express what a big deal this was to me. I was used to evaluating patients expertly, quickly processing the medical data to come up with a diagnosis and course of treatment. Now my brain was like mud—it just wouldn't respond. The able and astute Dr. Fox was nowhere to be found.

When the senior resident, Dr. Allan Sniderman, walked in to check on the patient, I froze. "I was totally paralyzed with fear of my lack of confidence." I presented the case to him in what I said was a completely incompetent way. "The findings were so striking that my senior looked at me in a manner that said, 'You have really had it, fellow.'" Then he asked to see the X-ray and for my diagnosis. I squirmed, not having a clue and running symptoms through my mind: "pansystolic murmur, fever, pale, spleen . . ." Finally, I blurted out, "Bacterial endocarditis" in desperation, thinking that couldn't possibly be correct.

"He cleared his throat in disbelief and said, 'I think we'd better see the X-ray.'" It couldn't be located. I wrote, "How could they have misplaced the X-ray at such a strategic moment? They could very well, and they had. I gasped in disbelief because I did not know. I felt that my mind would disintegrate." As they searched for the X-ray, I went out of the room and sat down, dumbfounded. Gloria called just then and asked how I felt. "Terrible, I am really going off my rocker! It's time for me to see the psychiatrist. Dr. Heinz Lehman at the Douglas Hospital is the only psychiatrist I trust. I'll have Dr. Sniderman call you to discuss what to do about me."

We left it there and got off the phone. Dr. Sniderman came over and said he agreed with my findings. It felt like a ton of bricks being lifted off my shoulders. In the meantime, my brother Allen had called Gloria. After they finished speaking, she called me again. "I am fine, no psychiatrist necessary." And then I wrapped up my observation: "That is the end of the worst day of my life."

HERE WE GO AGAIN

There's a void in my memory about what happened the rest of that week, between December 13 and 20. I knew that my thoughts were confused and that I had trouble functioning. From various medical records, I gleaned that I'd heard normal street sounds as magnified and lost my ability to concentrate. I acted hyperactive and garrulous at times. Other times, familiar things seemed alien to me. Apparently, I reported feeling puzzled by the most insignificant things, such as walking from one room to another.

Suffice it to say it wasn't a good week. My health problems were worsening, and I seemed to be descending into psychosis. On December 20, exactly a week after I was discharged from MNH, I was readmitted for what would be a four-day stay. My memories of this hospitalization are almost nonexistent. The discharge summary says I was admitted due to anxiety and memory impairment. The admission findings, which came from Dr. McNaughton, noted that I'd been discharged from MNH on December 13 after my first stay: *Soon after leaving the hospital, he seemed to have developed overt symptoms of anxiety, feelings of insecurity and even panic, and was very depressed. Repeated daily neurological examinations on December 17, 18 and 19 were normal. He then began to complain that he could not think clearly and noted gaps in memory, which made him feel he was having petit mal attacks. He was, therefore, readmitted on December 20 for further observation.* ("Petit mal" is the old name for the type of seizures now known as focal seizures. They occur in a single location in one brain hemisphere.)

The neurological exam findings were mostly normal. The doctor reported a tendency for me to hold the fingers of my left hand in odd positions compared to the right. And with my left hand there was a slight impairment of what's called stereognosis, which they tested by having me feel and hold coins. Stereognosis is the tactile ability to perceive the characteristics of an object, such as shape, by feeling it.

Lab tests showed an "acute lymphocytic reaction," meaning they found elevated lymphocytes in my cerebrospinal fluid, indicating inflammation or infection in the brain. They ran an EEG to measure the electrical activity in my brain and found some abnormal activity in the right hemisphere. The right side of the brain is responsible for movement and activity on the left side of the body.

While hospitalized, I was given a couple more medications to add to my existing regimen of the anti-seizure drugs Dilantin and phenobarbital. Doctors put me on chlordiazepoxide, which was then known under its brand name, Librium. This is an anti-anxiety drug in the benzodiazepine class, like Valium. In addition, I was prescribed Largactil (chlorpromazine), an antipsychotic that also was marketed back then under the name Thorazine.

After four days of tests and treatment, I was discharged from MNH. But this time, I wasn't going home. They were transferring me to a psychiatric hospital, AMI. Under the heading "Consultations," the MNH discharge report said, *Patient was seen by Dr. Lipowski, who felt that the patient's psychological disturbances were secondary to an organic brain disease, possibly an encephalitis, and advised a transfer to the Allan Memorial Institute.*

The term "organic brain disease" was used to describe a condition caused by a recognizable disease process, such as viral encephalitis, that was causing my mental health symptoms. That's as distinguished from a functional disorder of the brain with no identifiable cause, such as with many cases of schizophrenia.

My discharge diagnosis remained suspected viral encephalitis. On Christmas Eve, 1968, I was transferred to the psychiatric intensive care unit of AMI. My difficult journey was about to get longer and harder. It turns out I would be a psychiatric patient for almost two months.

CHAPTER 7
From the Inside Out

Before we get to the next stages of my medical misadventure—which took place on a psych ward—I want to pause to paint a picture of my illness from the personal and emotional angles.

Thus far, I've taken you through a roughly six-week timeline of my mysterious illness. It started with a brief aura episode with a flashing blue light and weaved through a trip to the ER, seizures, two hospitalizations, and a period in between when I made a disastrous effort to return to work and my confused mental state began to reveal signs of psychosis. We left off on Christmas Eve, 1968, the night doctors transferred me from MNH to AMI, a psychiatric hospital that would turn out to be my home for about the next two months.

For the most part, I've reported the progression of my illness through a medical lens—a chronological narrative, clinical in tone, and pieced together largely from fifty year's worth of professional medical records kept intact by the hospitals involved. They were crucial to help construct an accurate representation of what happened to me between November 1968 and February 1969. The records have also been enormously helpful in my quest to unearth the full details of the nature and course of my illness, treatment, and recovery. This is integral to the story, but it's an arm's-length view.

Just as there is far more to a Da Vinci masterpiece than its shapes, colors, and brush strokes, there is more to the tale of my illness than pharmaceutical dosages and abnormal electrical activity in the right parietal region of my brain. There's the story of the promising young physician who was suddenly thrown from a position of authority and landed on the receiving end of medical care feeling needy, helpless, and full of dread. There's also the story of the doctor's wife trying to navigate new and foreign terrain, juggling a job teaching teens with visits to the hospital and anxiously watching her husband's health rapidly decline. And there are parents, siblings, and friends, all trying to come to grips with the turmoil of a shocking new pins-and-needles reality.

Doctors can X-ray your skull and measure your brainwaves. They can't see what's in your mind and heart: your thoughts and dreams, your fears and aspirations, your bonds of love and friendship, or your deeply rooted psychic wounds. (Well, at least not yet. Who knows what science holds in store?)

To get a better image of the felt experience that won't show up on an EEG printout, we're going to dig back through that decrepit box I found in my basement in Wellesley after the pandemic hit in early 2020. The box contained contemporaneous personal accounts that I wrote mostly during the first part of my illness, prior to my stay at AMI. I've referred to these handwritten notes as a diary; actually, they seem a bit more random than one might expect from a diary.

My observations didn't chronicle the story with organized consistency. While many of them were undated, I was generally able to place them in time thanks to the fastidious record-keeping done in my old medical documents. Precision isn't as important in these personal notes because their value lies in providing a different camera angle rather than just adding to the volume of medical details. What emerges is a clear-cut view of my thoughts, moods, and opinions at the time. I'm presenting excerpts here in the format of a series of snapshots that are open for your own impressions and interpretations.

HOSPITAL LIFE

My first hospitalization at MNH ran from December 2–13, 1968. It's safe to say that I must have been somewhat shocked after the rapid transition from my normal state of energetic vitality to being confined in hospital with a mystery condition. I wasn't totally oblivious, though, given how I perked up to check out the singing nurses spreading Christmas cheer on the ward. It's interesting the way these two paragraphs pertaining to the exclusively female nurses are juxtaposed—a light-hearted note followed by a graphic description of nurses taking my temperature that's both morose and comical in nature:

> I must interrupt my writing to describe the group of well-dressed, pretty student nurses who are caroling. They are somewhat uncertain of exactly what they are to do and feel a little conspicuous standing in the middle of the ward, drawling out "Silent Night" in a not quite perfect harmony. However, they are quite cute and are doing what they are supposed to do. They fit their image and are doing a good deed.
>
> The nurses on average have been very pleasant, with the exception of their rectal thermometers. These instruments of torture have a peculiar cold, oozing feeling as they slide between the buttocks into the anal canal. While they rest quietly for three min-

utes, they are not bothersome. However, the mere knowledge of their presence causes discomfort. Finally, the moment of truth, and this grease-slimed heat projectile slips rapidly out, the buttocks slapping rapidly closed behind. A sigh of relief follows.

THE ANSWER TO LIFE

By December 10, I'd been in the hospital for more than a week and seemed to be doing some deep thinking, reflecting on the meaning and purpose of my life and career choice. My assumption that I would even have a future beyond the hospital walls indicates some underlying optimism about my recovery. If you recall, after I proposed to Gloria, I warned her that our financial prospects might be limited by my preference at that time to focus on pharmacological research rather than developing a lucrative medical practice. It seems my illness made me reconsider:

What is the answer to life for a physician? There are two basic choices:

1. *A life totally and fully selflessly devoted to a profession. This means a poor family life, a great deal of tension to produce, and competition for positions and grants. The obvious advantages are a certain contribution to the scientific knowledge in medicine and a feeling of accomplishment and recognition.*

2. *A life consisting of a fashionable practice in medicine, with a good income [and] respect in [the] community. If one works properly (e.g., in group practice), there is a good family life. One can enjoy family life and other finer things. Disadvantage: obscurity, no contribution to*

scientific knowledge. There is appreciation of patients and practice.

How to choose between two pathways? This is difficult. Until the time of my illness, my choice was made for the first pathway. However, during a few days in which I felt that my life might be over in the next year, I began to look at myself. What had I done in my life? A twenty-four-year-old physician, married with a beautiful, loving wife. Some good potential in the usual well-trodden pathways of medicine, an intellectual idiot in fields outside of medicine and an enjoyment, but no appreciation or understanding of the arts.

REACTION OF DOCTORS

My hospitalization represented a major role reversal for me. In the blink of an eye, I lost the leader's mindset and went from being a doctor in charge to a dependent patient whose daily life was now entirely planned and structured by others:

Sympathy from your professional confreres is great. They know it could happen to anyone, it just happened to be me. Everyone is shocked and hopes for the best. These kinds of episodes show that unfortunately doctors themselves are only human and are subject to the various disorders that they themselves treat.

This is one of the great burdens of the medical profession. Doctors study, discover, and treat, always knowing they themselves may fall victims to the same interesting secrets. The doctor solves this problem by denying this will ever happen to him. In other words, the doctor defends himself by giving himself a feeling of immortality. He will admit that he can get the illness, but deep down he really believes it cannot happen to him.

When a doctor becomes ill, then everyone is shocked. For a time, their defense of immortality is shattered by the living evidence of its falsity. Everyone is frightened because they realize it could have been them. But after a time, and time heals all, everything is forgotten.

It is said that man turns to his God when one is faced with death. For a few days I firmly believed that I had a brain tumor growing and that probably I would live one year.

HYPERVENTILATION

Normally, you breathe in air filled with oxygen that's absorbed into your blood, then you exhale carbon dioxide as a waste product. Hyperventilation describes the condition when someone exhales too much carbon dioxide in rapid, deep breaths. It can lead to low levels of carbon dioxide in the blood and resulting symptoms. A number of things can cause hyperventilation; the most common is anxiety or panic. In the movies or on TV, you've probably seen a freaked-out character breathe into a small paper bag when hyperventilating. The bag catches the carbon dioxide, which goes back into the body and helps restore the right balance with oxygen.

This note was dated December 11, 1968, two days prior to my discharge. I'd been given an EEG to measure my brain's electrical activity, during which doctors induced me to hyperventilate, something that enhances the results when looking for abnormalities from seizures or epilepsy. As a doctor, I had a thorough understanding of what happens during hyperventilation, so I was able to "keep calm and carry on," methodically observing my own responses:

This is an amusing experience for someone who understands what is happening and is consequently unafraid. After breathing deeply in and out through the mouth, the first sensation is one of dryness. This is followed a half minute later by a pulling feeling about the mouth, which goes on to a tingling sensation. As one continues at the end of two to two and a half minutes, the fingers feel odd and tingle if they are moved. When I stopped hyperventilating after three minutes, then there was the onset of a cold feeling with shivering all over. This shivering continued for about five minutes. The tingling of the mouth, fingers, and toes disappeared in about one minute. Soon all was well again, please note I did not feel dizzy.

PNEUMOGRAMS MAY BE FUN; DON'T ASK ME HOW

Pneumogram is a shorthand term for pneumoencephalo-gram, that super-unpleasant diagnostic procedure used in my case to look for possible brain tumors or scarring that might have caused my seizures. No longer in use today and replaced by other imaging methods such as the CT scan,[4] the procedure involved puncturing a patient's lower spine to drain the cerebrospinal fluid from around the brain, then injecting air to replace the fluid. That created more optimal photographic conditions for taking X-rays of the head. Many people preferred to have a general anesthetic so they could be completely out during the pneumoencephalogram.

My note gives a vivid and accurate description of what I endured during the procedure and its aftermath. To clarify a few points, "CNS" stands for central nervous system, which

---

[4.] J.D. Howell. The CT scan after 50 years-Continuity and change. New Eng. J Med 2021;385: 104-5.

is the brain and spinal cord. "IM" means intramuscular injection—into the muscles, as contrasted with intravenous, or in the veins. Librium and Valium are both sedatives in the benzodiazepine class, but Librium doesn't last as long in the system, making it a much poorer substitute for a general anesthetic than Valium:

> *The pneumogram (Pneumoencephalogram) is reputed to be one of the most uncomfortable tests that the medical profession has to offer. I have not had many tests, but I can vouch that it is a rather uncomfortable procedure (understatement). Do not let anyone ever tell you it is not too bad—it is terrible. My extensive experience includes one episode. I must point out that as a physician undergoing a CNS investigation, my friends wished to spare me the discomfort of the procedure and arranged a general anesthetic. The anesthetist asked my opinion about one hour before blast-off time, and I stated that it would be fine if all the systems were go without a general anesthetic.*
>
> *Unfortunately, my pre-medication was left to the radiologist whose knowledge of medications is as expected; not adequate. He generously prescribed 20 mg of IM Valium, which probably would have made me quite sleepy. However, when no Valium could be found, he settled for 20 mg of IM Librium, the effectiveness of which I need not discuss. He topped off this little cocktail with some atropine, which successfully dried my mouth.*
>
> *Now, with decisions to go ahead with the pneumogram made and the anesthetic problem dealt with, everything was ready except, oops, no one could find the nurse. She was that fine specimen of a grey-*

haired bitch who had patted my head earlier in the day and said that "You wouldn't give too much trouble." Now my back was bared as I lean over the special wooden stand for my arms, and my head is edged forward into the X-ray machine. "This is the time I tell my patients that this is my first try," I joked. "I have not done one for nineteen years." The radiologist returns. Then, the first poke of the needle, firmly, and then no pain. After a few minutes, there was a sharp pain in my back, a tingle in my right foot and toes. "Nice clear fluid, so far so good." The first little bit of air gives a small amount of pressure over the back of the head. "If this is what it is like, what a laugh. How could anyone complain about this?" I thought to myself.

Amusement was very short lived with the continued injection of air; I noted a flash of dull pain in my back. Then, my head began to feel like it was being compressed by a great weight. The pain was excruciating. I felt very ashamed to be groaning, but it first kept coming uncontrolled. I pushed on my head, pulled my hair, but the constant excruciating feeling just continued. Agonizing moments were worsened by my movements.

Finally, all the X-rays were taken, concluded to be normal, and I was returned to my room. I clung tightly to the cold washcloth on my forehead. I am not certain it helped or not, but it was distracting. When I returned to my room, all my family were conscientiously present to pay their respects. Unfortunately, the one person I wanted to see, my wife, was hurrying as fast as she could from teaching and was not yet present. I kicked everyone out and asked for a codeine injection. At last, my wife arrived. I asked to close the door, and she put her arms around me so I could cry.

After a few hours I was considerably improved, in spite of the constant taking of blood pressure policy and, worst of all, the flashlight in the eye, to test [my] pupillary response. This latter procedure is rather annoying, especially as it intensifies a terrible headache.

The next morning, I considered that I might sit up prematurely. The following were under consideration:

A. *One is supposed to stay flat on the back for thirty-six hours*

B. *It took forty-five minutes to pass urine into the damn bottle. I think that I unkinked my penis to get things started*

C. *Bedpan*

I took my chances and sat up slowly, prepared for the worst. Thank goodness nothing happened except for the occurrence of a minor headache. I breathed a sigh of relief and continued my usual hospital activities.

EMOTIONAL RESPONSE

I wrote this note on December 13, the day of my discharge from my first MNH hospitalization. I was in the middle of a glucose tolerance test for blood sugar levels that's used to check for diabetes. You have to fast for some extended period before the test and then drink a nauseatingly sweet glucose concoction. Then they periodically draw blood to see how effectively your body is producing the hormone insulin to process the sugar. The venipuncture I mention in my note refers to them puncturing a vein in my arm to take blood samples:

> *Although this is a wholly inadequate test, the medical profession is committed to follow things through to the bitter end. Ironically, I despise venipunctures, and my grand finale is a glucose tolerance test with nine venipunctures. Actually, the minimum now becomes eleven because the technician already missed twice. Five down, six to go.*
>
> *My performance last night is rather interesting; everything was fine. Then, I began to think that events have turned out very well—too well. People have been extremely pleasant to me—too pleasant. Then, I began to wonder why no one opposed my desire to return to work three days after leaving the hospital. Immediately after each test, I was told everything is perfectly normal. Putting all these facts together, I began to feel that maybe everyone was fooling me and trying to tell me that all was well although I am dying from a brain tumor. While I was thinking this, I realized it was ridiculous and that I was becoming paranoid.*
>
> *Trying to be objective, picture a twenty-five-year-old resident with a young wife who suddenly is found to have a brain tumor. Will they tell him? I was not certain. Certainly, I would know that if I have a tumor or not, you have to know where you stand!*
>
> *With my brain in a whirl, I phoned my wife. After explaining my crazy thinking that I had, she reassured me that our stories corresponded exactly. Sobbing during the conversation (something I can only do with my wife), I continued*

crying for a few minutes. A great feeling of tired-
ness came over me, and all the sobs racking my
body subsided. I said goodnight, put the phone
down, rolled over, and went to sleep.

BABY VS. EUROPE

It's not entirely clear exactly when I wrote this note. I suspect it was soon after my December 13 discharge from MNH. I had been accepted into a postdoctoral fellowship program at Duke University in Durham, North Carolina. It would be the summer or fall after my illness and follow my two years of internship and residency at the various hospitals connected with McGill in Montreal. I initially thought the program would start in September, giving us a couple of months before we had to move to the States.

My Duke fellowship would involve doing research in the laboratory of Dr. James B. Wyngaarden, the renowned chair of the Department of Medicine at Duke. Dr. Wyngaarden would later be appointed by President Ronald Reagan to serve as Director of the National Institutes of Health. I was thrilled to be working in his lab as part of a unique training program teaching physicians how to conduct laboratory research. To fund my work, I was awarded a two-year grant from the Medical Research Council of Canada.

> *Last night I received a letter from Dr. Wyngaarden,*
> *my boss in Durham, NC. He congratulated me on*
> *my grant and stated that I would [be]starting work*
> *in the beginning of July. My wife is very disap-*
> *pointed, for we had been planning a trip to Europe*
> *for the summer. I myself am anxious to go.*
>
> *But now I must remember I really want my wife*
> *to have a baby. The reason is simple: My illness is*
> *undiagnosed at the present time, and no one knows*

what the outcome will be. Everyone is optimistic; so am I. Being realistic, I may have an illness which will cause my deterioration. Therefore, in order to ensure some form of contribution, I feel a necessity to have a baby.

This is a simple, primitive desire of any man. He wants to leave something in the world afterwards. If the man is realistic, he knows that his existence in this world really only matters to a few people: those of his immediate family. They are the only ones who will come to remember him, and this they will not do conscientiously. With the passing of time and the immediate family, memories of the person are absolutely forgotten. He becomes a statistic in his country's demographic surveys. His tombstone is copied in the usual manner by the man doing his job.

This has been the fate of the majority of people except those who have been in major political office or those who have made gigantic contributions to their particular fields. Therefore, to leave children in the world after a person dies is a real contribution to his living memory. The children represent a partial embodiment of what he once was.

To leave a child is adequate, even better is to leave a child and a name, for this enhances the memory of the person. It is obvious that a firstborn son is the ideal to accomplish all these goals. This is why the firstborn son has always been the privileged one in many civilizations. That is simply why I want to have a baby, and I hope the child is a healthy, normal boy. This is selfish, but that is the way people are. We are important really only to ourselves. No one else aside from our immediate family cares.

All my personal observations excerpted above were written before my second hospitalization at Montreal Neurological. The collection in my basement contained only one further note, dated mid-February, towards the end of my extended stay at the AMI. We'll take a look at that account in the context of the discussion of my wild and woolly time at the psych hospital.

CHAPTER 8
PICU-Boo!

*All I want to do is come back to reality and exit
from my little world of terror and hallucinations.*

My second admission to MNH lasted four days, ending
with my transfer—on a stretcher—to AMI on December 24,
1968. Why? On top of the original symptoms of the aura and
seizures, I had developed psychiatric symptoms that were getting worse, such as confusion, disorientation, and anxiety.

These symptoms began to exhibit themselves as more
than just hints when I went home after my first MNH stay.
Every day brought new bits of evidence that I was losing my
grip on reality, whether that was hearing noises amplified or
finding powerful revelations in a children's book. I struggled
to relate to the world around me in the ways I always had
and to resume my pre-illness life. But my brain wasn't properly processing the information that came through the sense
gates, making it hard for me to recognize what was normal,
what was real.

Round two at MNH was for anxiety and memory impairment. The AMI admissions report by Dr. Guttman said I'd
been transferred from MNH due to "increasingly bizarre
behavior." During an exam at MNH the day before I was
transferred, I asserted that everyone around me was stupid.

On examination at AMI, Dr. Guttman listed her diagnostic impression as "acute schizophrenic reaction."

Schizophrenia causes bizarre thinking, strong or inappropriate feelings, and loss of interest in life. Dr. Guttman didn't diagnose me with functional (no identifiable cause) schizophrenia. Instead, she, and most of my doctors, thought I had an organic illness, such as viral encephalitis, that was causing my psychiatric symptoms. Functional schizophrenia might last forever. An acute schizophrenic reaction might go away when the underlying condition is resolved. Luckily, that's what happened to me—eventually. At this point, all was still cloaked in mystery.

The doctors at MNH were flummoxed enough about my condition to call for a psychiatric consultation. They brought in Dr. Z. J. Lipowski, a highly respected psychiatrist who was chief of the psychiatric consultation service at RVH, associate professor of psychiatry at McGill, and associate psychiatrist at AMI. It was on Dr. Lipowski's recommendation that I was transferred to AMI.

I arrived on December 24 and stayed about eight weeks, on two wards. For the first three and a half weeks, my home was the psychiatric intensive care unit (PICU). In a medical hospital, the sickest patients, those who need critical, sometimes one-on-one care, go to the ICU. Similarly, psychiatric hospital patients with the most extreme mental symptoms and illnesses go to the PICU, where they can be closely watched and provided with the level of care they need.

I make it sound so clinical, almost sterile. It was anything but! Imagine suddenly being plucked out of your daily routine and dropped into a community of strangers, where the residents all suffer mental problems, many with weird manifestations, and you're not exactly lucid yourself. I'm sure the day I strolled out to the nurses' station in the altogether, it was just another eye-roller for the staff, something they'd seen dozens of times before. For me, judging by what I wrote, life on the PICU was a wretched experience, compounded by my confusion, divorce from familiar surroundings, and medication side effects.

WELCOME TO THE FUNNY FARM —IT'S NO LAUGHING MATTER

The personal accounts I wrote during my illness contain only one entry after mid-December 1968, and that one poses a puzzle. It comprises a series of short commentaries, each generally distinct from the other. My memory of those two months at AMI is almost a complete void, providing no help in contextualizing these personal notes. Fortunately, I have other reliable sources to fill in the gaps, including extensive medical records. They contain doctors' reports and bedside notes by nurses who were experts in documenting the physical condition and behavior of psychiatric patients. The interviews I conducted in 2020 clarified things even more.

In reviewing the medical notes, I noticed that the date on the sole personal account I wrote at AMI didn't correspond with the events it described—even if they were figments of my psychotic imagination. My note bears the date February 12, 1969, which was just a week before my final discharge. By then, I was well on my way to recovery. The disoriented nature of my writings points to my PICU stay, when my physical and behavioral symptoms were the most pronounced.

A key feature of my psychosis was forgetfulness of dates and timelines, particularly regarding my own illness. It's possible I thought it was February in January. Or maybe I wrote scattered notes as they happened and collected them all together under the February 12, 1969, umbrella. They're written in the past tense, lending credence to the February date. Yet my memory was so impaired, I don't know how I would've remembered details of events that took place weeks earlier.

The questions on the timing of my notes may never be answered. Nevertheless, the notes are important to include here since they're the only first-person accounts I have of my two months as a psych patient. While some of my comments are obviously mistaken, they also provide a rare glimpse into the deluded mind of someone whose mental faculties have broken down. I've added explanations and supporting materials to help bring the events into sharper focus.

They rolled me into the PICU at 5 p.m. on Christmas Eve, accompanied by my wife, brother, and father, who all must have been terribly upset to see me so ill. According to the very first nurse's bedside note from AMI, I came in on a stretcher and seemed very drowsy. I wrote a comment about my last couple of hours at MNH, followed by another that appears to describe an ambulance ride and getting settled into a double room in the PICU:

> A doctor interviewed me and said, "I can help you." One hour later, the nurse entered, needle in hand, ready to strike my butt. Then, a stretcher carried me away from the neurological hospital to the psychiatric hospital.
>
> Sirens whirring, I was carried up and [had] my blood pressure taken. A panicking nurse took it and cried, "It's falling!" Someone else was trying to take my temperature with a thermometer in the left armpit, an inaccurate maneuver long discarded. It almost broke and I was fighting. Then, upstairs in a ward, a bed with clean sheets. Two hours later, ouch, another

nurse with a needle in hand and pills also, six at a
time are given.

The nurse wrote that about ninety minutes after my arrival, *He got out of bed and walked to the hall, but he suddenly faced the wall and said that he could not walk anymore, that his legs were weak, and that he could not see.* They helped me back to bed, where I was given a shot of Largactil and fell asleep.

I want to discuss Largactil for a moment, as it plays a big role in this part of my story. The generic name is chlorpromazine, which is also marketed under the brand name Thorazine. In use for about seventy years now, chlorpromazine was a first-generation antipsychotic drug. It falls into a class of antipsychotics called phenothiazines. These drugs were groundbreaking in treating symptoms of schizophrenia, bipolar disorder, and other conditions. I'm convinced they helped me. But they do have significant negative side effects.

For much of the time I was on Largactil, I also took another phenothiazine called Stelazine, which treats symptoms of schizophrenia and anxiety. Combining Stelazine and Largactil can increase the side effects. Without going too deep in the weeds here, phenothiazines reduce levels of the brain hormone dopamine, which is involved with many body functions, including pleasure, movement, motivation, learning, attention, mood, digestion, blood flow, and more. Low dopamine is associated with symptoms of Parkinson's disease. When these same symptoms are produced by conditions other than Parkinson's, they're sometimes called parkinsonism.

This is just a partial list of potential side effects of phenothiazines:

- A shuffling walk
- Slow, odd, or uncontrollable body movements
- Feeling dizzy or unsteady, balance problems, falling

- Confusion
- Agitation, restlessness, nervousness
- A blank expression
- Difficulty urinating
- Constipation
- Difficulty falling sleep or staying asleep
- Dry mouth
- Skin rash, itching
- Abdominal cramps

Many of these side effects are featured prominently in my personal notes.

> *Phenothiazines are an experience. They lead to total immobilization. Shuffling walk is an experience with a tremor and obvious grotesque arm movements. Mouth is dry and one must drink all the time. The urine does not come as desired and has to be thought about. Urinary retention is extremely uncomfortable. A full bladder and pressure, but no drop of that golden liquid. Constipation set in, bringing pressure to the abdomen. If the bowel movement is not good, the day is not good. What else is as satisfying as a good shit? A rash on the palms of the hands and the soles of the feet sets in with itchiness. What a way to live. Then, some more pills to counteract the side effects of the other pills. There is secrecy and oblivion concerning your condition. There is no information, how long, or why. The diagnosis is not clear. Psychiatrists say "encephalitis." The neurologist observes one seizure and other tests are normal except for a few cells in the cerebral spinal fluid.*

The medical records contain numerous reports that illustrate the side effects I experienced. On December 25, my first full day on the PICU, a nurse wrote that I was very slow to answer questions. I would hesitate and say, "I don't understand." I needed verbal directions and would stare at the person speaking to me for a long time. The note continued, *Appears vague and uncoordinated, i.e., unable to tie his shoes. He says "I can't see things right. I feel as though I'm in a dream."*

The next day, December 26, I was up at 6 a.m. and went to the dayroom, where I sat and stared at the wall, asking, "What happened to reality? I don't understand it." I was unable to walk back to my room on my own. The nurse's note said, when assisted, left one arm in a raised position for at least two minutes—arm had been resting on nurse's shoulder. Legs appeared very rigid. Was unable to put them in bed unassisted while sitting on bedside. My body didn't feel right, and it worried me. "It's all wrong. It's crooked!" I thought. Staff said I couldn't communicate verbally and that I needed help with basic hygiene and eating. I was a mess!

Midnight on December 27 found me standing in my room doing toe-touch exercises. Unable to sleep, I showed up later at the nurses' station, asking for the doctor: "I want to know the dosage of my Largactil. It causes urethral spasms." I went back to my room, and the nurses' note says they later heard me shouting. When attendant entered, patient was lying on the floor with knees drawn up, screaming, "My bladder is twisted!" Apparently, I told them I wanted to see whether the floor was more comfortable than the bed. In a report dated December 29, Dr. Lowy referred to this as an example of "somatic delusions." In addition to complaining that the Largactil had twisted my bladder, I thought my blood pressure cuff was stuck under my skin.

A couple of times, I just seemed to slide to the floor from a standing or sitting position, like I was melting. That matches the drug side effects. One such incident took place on

December 27: *Stood by the nursing station, his eyes closed and swaying. When asked to open his eyes, he began to really sway and sank to the floor with a nurse and an attendant holding onto him.*

December 28 was a rough day. I'd been awake most of that night, jumping over my bed rails to go look at calendars in the dayroom, saying I needed to study for my work in North Carolina. I was restless all day: *Has been speaking very rapidly and quite incoherently for long periods. Misperceiving objects in his environment, i.e., thought the line between two tables was a stick and that a round ashtray was a halo.* Fifteen minutes after I received a shot of Largactil, I thought there had been an accident and put a bunch of chairs in the hallway to create a roadblock. Earlier, I had refused my oral meds and started yelling, "You're making me crazy!"

When my parents came to visit in the afternoon of December 28, I was rational. Afterwards, I was seen talking to a woman named Gigi Perrault. Now, Gigi is Gloria's nickname, but her maiden name was nothing like Perrault, who wasn't actually there. I was hallucinating. They gave me more Largactil; no change. I made random, inexplicable comments, such as, "John they have guns now," "Things are very tense, but they do seem to be easing up a little," and "He worked at security yesterday."

They kept giving me more Largactil, but I slept very poorly that night. The nurses say I was having auditory and visual hallucinations. I thought I was driving a car and said, "Look at all the policemen." Around 2 a.m. on December 29, they heard a cry and a thump and found me face down on the floor near the foot of my bed, entangled in my bedsheets. After that, a staff member stayed with me until I finally fell asleep at 5 a.m.

I refused my scheduled pills frequently, sometimes throwing them on the floor. In the TV room, I thought—mistakenly—that

I had voided in the room. I jumped up and down and pointed my finger at the wall. Later that night, the nurse wrote that I was in the lounge, stamping my feet with my right hand raised in the air. When asked what I was doing, I responded, "I'm walking to hell." The note concludes, *Returned at 10:30 p.m.* Returned from hell? Perhaps a stab at humor by the nurse, in a mostly humorless environment.

Interviews done with friends and family in 2020 shed more light. My sister and brother-in-law, Rosanne and Steve Ain, came to visit early in my AMI stay. Rosanne said, "The thing we both remember is you didn't know left from right and you were flipping your feet over each other back and forth so I could figure out which is your left and which is your right foot." Steve explained why this was so striking: "It was bizarre that here you were, a physician, a gold medal medicine student, and you didn't know your left from your right!" Yes, bizarre indeed.

Lenny Diamond says he found me robotic and lacking emotion. Lenny played chess with me in the hospital. When the quality of my game was improving, he could tell that my disease state was improving. He clearly remembers my shuffling walk and says he was relieved to learn it was a side effect and not a symptom of my illness.

My parkinsonian symptoms were very hard on Gloria. She recalls the way I shuffled my feet and had to inch backwards to sit in a chair. When I finally came home from the hospital, she said, "I had to throw out those slippers because I couldn't stand the sound of them." Someone had given me Brut after-shave lotion, and to that she said, "Uh-uh, throwing that one out too! I don't want any memories of the hospital."

When I interviewed my friend Arnie, he had gone on to pile up achievements in an illustrious medical career filled with honors and recognition. Ultimately becoming

Dean of the Faculty of Medicine and Vice Provost for Health Care Institutions at University of Toronto Medical School, Arnie was honored for his major career accomplishments by being appointed as a member of the Order of Canada. Despite such a busy life, he had some storage space in his memory banks for some anecdotes about his many visits to me at AMI, and we shared some laughs.

In a comical role reversal, Arnie related one wacky story in my voice, as I had told it to him: "Last night, around midnight, Dr. McNaughton came to my room and took me to the basement of the MNH. His mother was buried there and was in a coffin. Her body was surrounded by candles, and Dr. McNaughton made me pray to her." Then Arnie said to me, "Irving, that can't be true," and I responded, "I know! I know it can't be true!" Dr. Lowy suggested that at times I was having dreams that I could not distinguish from reality. Sounds like a good theory in this case.

Arnie also recalls me telling him the slipper vomit story that I wrote about in my personal account, which involved my PICU roommate, an Egyptian man named Balikian. Arnie never thought the story was true, though he did find it interesting: "Beside me quietly rested an Egyptian man, Balikian. His feet were big, his shoes were gigantic, but he was not tall. [He was] a fine man with a pipe and his lady to give him a manicure. His fancy dinner jacket was beautiful. But the next morning he vomited on my slippers. What a mess and stink!"

WHAT HAPPENED TO REALITY?

It's a peculiar feeling reading what I wrote in the middle of such turbulent times, my memory a blank. I can recognize very little of my youthful self. Mostly I feel far removed. At the same time, my heart goes out to that young man (and others in the same boat) for the suffering and indignities he endured and the way he kept grasping for familiar pieces of his life, hoping to make sense of an alien landscape. What follows are sections of my notes that show how painful it often was:

> *Being in a psychiatric ward is an unfortunate experience. The intensive care unit was a nightmare with injections and restricted movement. Pills are doled out and forced down the throat. Dr. Fox wants to go back to work, but how can a sick doctor take care of ill patients? Who do you speak to penned in a two-roomed bedroom with a curtain for a door? A person cannot even shit or shower in comfort. How does one escape? Stuck alone, sleepy with parkinsonism. Nighttime was always scary. The nurses have the right to give injections as necessary. Wow, what a sore bum! For days afterwards, I could only stand; sitting was an ordeal. What is intensive care? This means constant watching. A man cannot crap without somebody listening to the gas and commenting on the fumes. No peace for the suffering in this world.*
>
> *A myriad of psychiatrists in their suits passed by. "How are you today? How are you feeling?" "I have been working too hard and two seizures struck me." They all look at me queerly and nod their heads. All I want to do is come back to reality [and] exit from my little world of terror and hallucinations.*

Elsewhere, I wrote that Gloria and my parents visited every day. I'm sure I found comfort in believing that. Gloria remembers otherwise. She lived with my parents while I was ill. They would alternate visiting days; she came one day and my parents the next. Whoever's turn it was would go home to provide a full report, and they'd all sit and debate my progress.

> *Eat, drink, sleep, take pills, tremble, and not walk are the activities that occupy the time. Blood pressure is taken at breakfast, lunch, supper, and bedtime. How is it? A big secret. The patient is not allowed to know. Then, visiting hours bring my wife to me. Faithfully she comes every night with my parents, bringing the evening luscious apple. But there is no privacy to talk, kiss, and hold each other close.*
>
> *When do you go home? When are you transferred to another ward where there are more privileges? Playing cards all day long is boring. Crazy 8's was the dominant game. It does not require much thought, especially for those who are unable to concentrate.*

The bedside note of January 4 says I came to the office several times around breakfast time asking for my uniform so I could go to work. When I would realize that wasn't happening, I would go take a shower—with supervision, of course—after complaining that the clean towels looked dirty. The report said, *Quite pleased when he could go for a walk. Went to dress and said his clothes were not his and thought his own had been stolen. Later said he just didn't feel like a walk just yet.* I may have been referencing the stolen clothes when I wrote this entry:

> *In addition, everyday possessions and money disappear. There is a loss of ability to concentrate with mind wandering. Existence becomes so futile with no answers to the questions.*

My next comment has a different perspective on that walk outside. My note makes it look like I took the walk, but the nurse indicates I didn't. I was still confused about dates and places, because this note mentions an incident during an EEG that probably occurred back on December 23 at MNH:

> *Getting dressed was indeed a great production with special permission required from the doctor who, of course, is unreachable. The residents and nurses have no authority to call or cancel those orders. A walk outside was a great step. The fantastic outdoors with 100 inches of snow hiding cars, sparkling, blowing, and glittering with the sun shining. Schizophrenic symptoms are frightening. Loud voices, loud noises, people talking when nobody is present. One day while taking an electroencephalogram, in order to save the world, I stood up and shouted, "You're all stupid!" A warning was necessary for them to stop helping.*

On January 6, after being awake most of the night, I was up early. Apparently, I was quite upset because I'd been incontinent, but staff calmed me down, changed my linens, and I got back into bed. Not for long. I soon marched out to the nurses' station, stark naked, declaring, "I seem to have lost my clothes, and I have to be on duty in a little while."

There are two notes in the medical records from a Dr. Martin, dated January 9 and 10, when I'd been on the PICU for more than two weeks. He felt my condition was essentially unchanged. At times I was reasonable and realistic, then I'd flip back to confused, anxious, and tense. The following day he wrote, He still shows thought disorder and lack of judgement when he keeps asking for his books, stating that he has to go back to work to take care of his patients.

My Largactil dose had been increased by 50 percent: mainly because two days ago I was restless, was becoming angry to the point where he tried to hit one of the attendants. It's not crystal clear from the records, but it seems that my outburst occurred after I'd tried to go to the visiting area where I thought my family was waiting. I reportedly became very agitated when I was told otherwise, shouting, "I don't believe you!" Based on what I said in my personal note, I may have tried to run to the visiting area to see for myself:

> *Running away down the maze of winding halls was one of my performances. Then, the attendant caught me, and I punched him and kicked and scratched, aiming for the testicles, but not reaching them. How did I get here?*

STEP DOWN FROM PICU

During the second week in January, I was still having quite a bit of confusion, disorganization, inappropriate behaviors, and medication side effects. Was I improving? That's not certain. I had my share of lucid moments, participated in therapy group, was able to feed myself, and was more animated in my interactions with others. It was a positive sign that one evening I was studying endocrinology, though the nurse reported that I appeared to be explaining the subject matter *to a nonexistent body in the next chair.*

In a note written on January 13, Dr. Naiman said my mental status showed considerable fluctuation: *There are episodes during which he manifests hallucinations, delusions, and illusions.* But what seemed to stand out the most to Dr. Naiman was an increase in my trend towards depression. In a separate note on the same day, Dr. Martin wrote, *it seems that the patient is now acting more like a psychotic depressive.*

To stop that trend, Dr. Naiman wanted to start me on a tricyclic antidepressant called Elavil. A few doctors discussed the idea and cooked up a plan to safely introduce the new med. You see, there was a risk that starting me on Elavil to combat symptoms of depression might actually exacerbate my psychosis. They decided to increase my dosage of Largactil over a period of several days, hoping it would reduce my psychotic symptoms enough to offset any increase caused by the antidepressant. They had already started raising my Largactil doses, which were quite high compared to today's standards for the same drug. There was a risk of increasing side effects.

My doctors, however, were not all singing in the same key. Dr. Robert A. Cleghorn had examined me at AMI. His visit was an unusual occurrence since he was the chair of psychiatry at McGill University and a giant in the history of Canadian psychiatry. My medical records don't contain any reports directly from Dr. Cleghorn, but on January 14, Dr. Naiman wrote, *Dr. R. A. Cleghorn is in favor of diminishing medications*. My team of providers would discuss my case the next day. *In the meantime, plan to increase medications cancelled.*

The opinion of Dr. Cleghorn seemed to carry considerable weight around AMI. The increase in medications was not only cancelled but reversed, as they gradually reduced my dosages of Largactil. On January 16, Dr. Martin wrote that the Largactil increase had been stopped at 125 mg. t.i.d. (three times/day). He noted that I was somewhat less depressed and more aware of what was happening around me. The very next day, Dr. Martin saw more improvement, writing, *The patient appears to be better. He is more organized, more appropriate, and appears to be somewhat less depressed.* The Largactil had been reduced to 50 mg. t.i.d.

Dr. Naiman had arranged for my transfer, and on January 17, 1969, I left the psychiatric ICU and stepped down to a less intensive level of care in the regular psych ward known as North II. I was pretty happy about making that advance:

> *Then, the big day, when I transferred to a new ward, second in the Allan Memorial Hospital in a luxurious room.*

CHAPTER 9
The Bumpy Road to Recovery

My new room wasn't truly luxurious. But my digs on the North II psych ward of AMI must have given me at least a mental sense of spaciousness after suffering what I'd experienced as oppressiveness from constant surveillance and nonexistent privacy in the PICU.

I guess I was stringing together enough scattered periods of lucidity that my doctors thought I could be safely transferred to a regular ward in the psychiatric hospital. I wouldn't characterize this as steady improvement. It's better described as a series of slight to modest improvements that were countered by frequent symptomatic episodes.

Still, it's fair to say that the second half of January 1969 was a sort of midsection of my AMI hospitalization that marked a transition between the periods of serious illness and recovery. I'd been admitted to AMI on Christmas Eve, 1968, because of the worsening behaviors of my psychosis. I spent more than three weeks in the PICU, extremely sick and out of touch with reality most of the time. Only in the last few days before my transfer to North II on January 17,

1969, did I begin to show signs that maybe, just maybe, the worst was over.

Was that due to a change in the medication strategy of reducing, rather than increasing them? Was my illness running its course? Was it both? It's hard to know. What I can say is that even though I was still quite sick, the transfer to North II seemed to fuel my determination to get better. The doctors' reports and the nurses' bedside notes in this chapter span the period between my transfer off the PICU on January 17 and my February 19 discharge. They cover my bouts with ongoing symptoms and drug side effects, and they illustrate how my drive to return to my career and family life propelled me on the road to recovery. The nurses' bedside notes were signed with a first initial and last name only, sometimes illegibly. In quoting the nurses' bedside notes here, I've left off the names.

LIFE ON NORTH II

Before lunch on January 17, I arrived at my new ward, dressed in pajamas. If I was happy about leaving the PICU, the nurse couldn't tell, writing that I appeared tense and anxious, *with no facial expression and kept hands in one position, clasped on his lap.* I seemed interested when staff showed me around after lunch, but I was *perspiring quite a bit.* In addition, *Patient walks with a shuffle and arms in a constant position bent in front of him. Has been pacing the hall a bit and walking about sometimes aimlessly.* Later, while chatting with a group of patients and staff, I was asked how I wanted to be addressed. I answered, "Mister," and then corrected that to "Doctor." I said that would remind me I was a doctor, something I *was inclined to forget.* Sounds like I wanted to rebuild my sense of identity as a physician.

A bedside note of January 19 depicts a rough morning: *Arrived at breakfast table in an anxious state. Sat rigidly on edge of chair holding plate of toast in left hand and eating with right for at least three or four minutes before setting plate down on table. Appearance was disheveled. Spilt coffee into saucer and scattered crumbs all over place setting. On approach by staff, he was nervous and slightly disoriented. Asked twice in the half hour what the day and time was.*

A staff member suggested I try to allay my anxiety with a shower. I did so and returned within the hour, neatly dressed and relaxed. I was better, but not entirely right: *He continues to move in a robot-like manner and frequently perspires profusely.* Asked again later about what made me anxious, I said there was nothing specific, adding that I regretted not being able to spend more time with my wife.

The bedside note continued: *Then he stated almost mechanically, "I am a junior resident at the Royal Victoria Hospital," reintroducing himself to staff with whom he had previously worked. Said he was causing a lot of inconvenience to other residents who had worked with him and expressed fear of losing his research grant this summer in North Carolina. Said he had difficulty remembering he was still a patient and constantly seems to demand more of himself.*

Trouble arose later, according to the nurse's note: *During supper, started stuttering and moaning loudly at intervals. When returned to ward, it continued at two-to-three-minute intervals. Expressing fear about going crazy. Lucid between intervals of this behavior and conscious of what was happening. Would become more rigid, i.e., twitching of left side of face. At supper had illusion that plate was full of vomitus. Anxious with profuse diaphoresis. At 6:15 p.m., Largactil 50 mg IM given during these intervals.* (Diaphoresis is excessive, abnormal sweating and the IM after Largactil means it was given by intramuscular injection. I finally settled down by 7:00 p.m.

Largactil has many possible side effects, such as shuffling, odd body movements, agitation, blank expression, etc. Sweating like a horse is not among them. A week or so earlier, my doctors on the PICU had started increasing my doses in anticipation of starting me on an antidepressant. When McGill's Chief of Psychiatry opined that my medications should be reduced, the plan was stopped in its tracks. By January 16, my Largactil dosage had reached 125 mg. t.i.d. (three times a day) and was reduced to 50 mg. t.i.d. It was quite a dosage roller coaster inside of a week, though I doubt it was the cause of the moaning-and-groaning episodes.

Dr. Naiman addressed these episodes in his report of January 20, adding more details on the facial twitches: *The twitching involved the left side of his face from the eye to the lip. There was no mention of the forehead, and these episodes did not go on to generalized seizures. During these episodes the patient was unresponsive.*

He also wrote that a prior EEG of my brain *showed a disturbance over the right hemisphere.* Electrical disturbances on the brain's right side could conceivably cause twitching on the left side of my face. *It seems reasonably clear that this patient has some kind of focal cerebral disturbance.* So the moaning-and-groaning episodes were probably small seizures or seizure-like activity. But there's another twist: *With respect to the episode last night, it should be noted that, although he has been on Dilantin 100 mg. t.i.d. for some time, the phenobarb that he was also receiving was discontinued by me a few days ago as part of the general programme of reducing his total amount of medication, and consequently part of this activity may be a result of phenobarb withdrawal.*

Phenobarbital is a barbiturate drug I'd been taking to prevent seizures since my first hospitalization in early December. It works by slowing brain activity, and is habit-forming. The six or seven weeks I'd been on it isn't exactly long term, but I probably should have come off it gradually, not cold turkey. Abrupt withdrawal can cause seizures and other symptoms, possibly including diaphoresis.

Dr. Naiman felt I had some kind of neurological disorder that was creating the secondary psychiatric symptoms. He concluded his report saying it was puzzling that the shot of Largactil I received the evening before seemed to stop what he called the "epileptiform activity," meaning the seizure-like behavior. He was surprised because the drug has no known anti-seizure properties. *If anything, it is alleged to facilitate epileptiform activity.*

Dr. McNaughton did a detailed neurological exam the next day and found everything normal: *I have noted the report of periods of confusion, trembling, and twitching of left side of face—prefer not to resume treatment with phenobarbital unless there is stronger evidence of seizure activity.* He ordered an antibody titer, which is a blood test to look for signs of infection. He also ordered another lumbar puncture (a.k.a., spinal tap) to check my cerebrospinal fluid for evidence of infection or inflammation in the brain.

Over about the next ten days, I continued to have difficult periods that were gradually interspersed with stretches of normalcy in both my mindset and activities. A bedside note of January 21 says I was anxious and tense most of the day and became very agitated when I participated in a large group therapy session. My blood pressure fluctuated sharply: *Extremely anxious—stuttering, fumbling, both hands shaking visibly.*

Two days later, on January 23, I was happy about getting a haircut, and I knew the pharmaceutical names of my meds. The bedside note said I went to the coffee shop with another patient and staff, gossiping about RVH where I worked. I spent time reading with *fair concentration and minimal anxiety.* I had the spinal tap, which I tolerated well, and I rested quietly afterwards.

January 25 saw me staying in my room all day. I said I was studying, but the nurse who wrote that day's bedside note wasn't sure how well I could concentrate. My manner was described as stiff: *Unable to initiate a conversation or even carry a conversation with staff.* I felt better, saying I was ready to return to work. The note said I couldn't cope with certain visitors and didn't understand the implications of that with regard to my ability to cope with my job.

In the middle of the night on January 27, staff found me sitting on the side of my bed, saying there was something in the sheets. When they changed the bedding, I slept only fitfully, waking at 4 a.m., when I was described as "blocking in speech" in the nurse's note, which went on: *Quite anxious and agitated at this point, flicking his light switch off and on. Patient asked for a PRN—got very suspicious as to the kind of medication to be given to him. When a nurse approached with the injection, he told her he had just received one. Very rigid and shaking while injection being given—hands hanging in the air at his sides.* (PRN means "as needed.") Nurses were able to give me extra doses of Largactil at their discretion.

The note recounts that the trouble continued: *Patient became more confused and [was] hallucinating—saying that he was seeing things and then things would disappear. Began going in and out of his room—turning lights on and off, standing in the middle of his room staring. When walking, did so with stiff, propelled type of walk.* I remained agitated, with visual hallucinations. They gave me another dose of Largactil. The note said that at 10 a.m., *Continues to hallucinate. Staff's attempts to bring him back to reality increasingly difficult. Becomes very rigid, picking at sheets, talking of farms, boats, water.*

Despite this, when Dr. Naiman came in to see me that same morning, he reported I was "considerably improved and in good spirits." So, he decided to discontinue the Largactil entirely, without tapering the dose first. There was still a standing PRN order for Largactil. At the start of Dr. Naiman's visit, I seemed completely lucid, but then, *He began to talk about farming and stated that he was in a farmhouse.* I said that the female nurse who'd been at my bedside was a man with a male name. Dr. Naiman ordered an immediate EEG in the hope of seeing whether there were any differences in my brain's activity when I was in one of these confused states.

As the end of January approached, I grew more preoccupied with returning to work. A bedside note of January 29 said, *When asked how well he was, patient stated 75 percent, appeared downcast and tense. At this time spoke of thinking of himself too much. Where before he could lose himself in his work, spoke of difficulty in adjusting to this new situation. Quite tense and anxious during this time.* I opened up and spoke about my heavy workload before I had the flashing blue light and seizures. I talked about my two previous hospitalizations, my fear of having a brain tumor, and my great relief when I found out I didn't have one.

Later, I was even more candid, according to the same note: *Spoke of feeling lonely here. Feels rejected by his friends. Finally admitted to feeling angry and depressed. Accepted that these feelings of remorse are normal, but that he has difficulty accepting this as he never acknowledged them before.*

The analysis of my cerebrospinal fluid was finished. Dr. Naiman wrote, *the conclusion of the pathologist is this is a subsiding inflammatory reaction. It would seem that our initial diagnostic impression that this was a reaction secondary to some sort of encephalitis is confirmed by the spinal fluid findings.* The word "subsiding" brought hope that an end might be in sight. Dr. Naiman noted that I'd been on Valium, and since there had been no recurrence of acute psychiatric symptoms, he was going to start reducing the dosage.

THE HOME STRETCH

Starting at the end of January, the nurses' notes grew shorter and less frequent. They didn't need to write as much about the positives as they did about the problems. A January 31 note said I was *very spontaneous, socializing well.* I studied endocrinology, then went down to the gym and played basketball. On February 3, I spent most of the day in my room studying, breaking only when visitors came. I was trying to catch up with my missed work.

I studied a great deal but also took part in hospital programming. I actively engaged with others in a therapy group, and I attended poetry and art groups. All was not roses, however. On February 6, during art group, I said I was hearing voices and asked if a staff member was calling me.

The bedside note says that within ten minutes, I was no longer disoriented or delusional. That night, I was happy I'd be let out on a partial weekend pass, noting I was eager to be with my wife. The nurse wrote that I played ping-pong *and appeared quite bright, talking and laughing.*

On Monday, February 10, Dr. Naiman dismissed concerns about my hearing voices, noting *this kind of hallucination* was benign and *may safely be disregarded.* He said I'd done well over the weekend, when I'd gone out each day for a few hours. If all went smoothly during the week, I could spend the whole next weekend at home. Dr. Naiman wrote, I *do not propose to delve into this patient's psychopathology,* meaning I didn't need to have my head shrunk. If anything, *I think that he should be discharged as soon as possible.*

The same Monday, the nurse's note read, *Attended lecture at RVH with permission and returned grinning ear to ear—apparently, he had asked several questions at the lecture and several persons had inquired where he had been. This did not bother him. He said simply that he had been ill. Plans to go to another lecture on Wednesday.* Later, I went down to the gym with two other patients and said how much I'd enjoyed my weekend out and the lecture. I was eager to get off my medications and be done with the side effects.

On February 17, I did some studying in the morning, then attended film and art groups before heading off to join rounds at RVH. Dr. Naiman's note that day said I'd had a very good weekend out and they planned to discharge me in two days. They wanted me to take a ten-day holiday, then come see Dr. Naiman for an office visit before returning to work on limited duties, "under fairly close supervision."

The final, beautiful nurse's note from AMI was written on Wednesday, February 19: *Patient discharged at 10:30 a.m. Brother came to pick him up at hospital. Seemed quite bright and anxious to go home today.* I don't remember this, but I said, "Amen!" The discharge report listed all the tests, studies, and lab work, which found nothing strongly conclusive about what was wrong with me. They felt certain that the cause was not something psychiatric and that my mental symptoms were secondary to an organic brain disease, likely a viral encephalitis. Final diagnosis: *acute brain syndrome—etiology unknown.*

MEMORIES

There are a few more notable recollections from the friends and family members I interviewed in 2020. My friend Lenny Diamond is now retired in Toronto after a successful career as a periodontist. He's actually a relative now, having married Gloria's second cousin a few months after my discharge. Lenny wasn't too focused on the future or the question of whether I would recover: "I only thought of the present. Every day I saw you, I was hoping that it was the cure day." Still, Lenny admits he worried that I might lose my intellectual and cognitive abilities: "Well, I was happy you recovered because basically I loved you like a brother, and it was really a major concern because you were one of the brightest medical people that has ever come out of McGill and I said, 'Oh my god, I hope that this is not going to change as a result of this problem.' So, I was kind of relieved when you recovered."

Arnie Aberman says he always felt sure I'd recover. Not so of my younger brother Allan, a neuroradiologist. Allan recalls our strange, disjointed conversations when he visited. There was another patient named Fox, and I came up with the wacky idea of organizing a "Fox club." Allan just humored me, but he worried I might never recover. Once I did start to improve, he feared I might not gain back my full capacity and thought that might impact my career.

My sister and brother-in-law, Rosanne and Steve Ain are both retired and live in Toronto. Rosanne was a high school math teacher, and Steve was a renowned Jewish community organizer. They were very worried and uncertain about my prospects for recovery, according to Rosanne: "It was really hard because you were my older brother and you were a very successful student starting in a career, and we wondered if it would ever happen. So, it was very scary, but we were twenty-one, you know; we were really kids."

Whatever started this extraordinary three-month ordeal, Steve thinks it's remarkable how quickly my recovery began to almost cascade at the end of January: "I do remember when you were starting to get better, it came on very quickly . . . We had no understanding of it, but thank goodness you started to get better and it sort of accelerated. It was like you came back to normal and nothing had ever happened."

DR. ROBERT FORREST

I've mentioned that my memory of my time at AMI is a complete blank. I do have a wisp of a memory of a visit I had from a medical resident I didn't know. Someone had warned me to ignore him because he'd had status epilepticus, which may sometimes cause permanent brain damage. Status epilepticus refers to having more than one seizure in a five-minute period or having a single seizure lasting more than five minutes. Dr. Forrest had suffered problems similar to mine and believed his condition was caused by viral encephalitis.

Having been steered off paying Dr. Forrest any heed, plus being in a rather bad physical and mental state, I did wipe his visit out of my head. At least until, in 2020, I discovered a letter from him that I received soon after my discharge (JAR in the letter stands for junior assistant resident):

Dear Irving,

I hope you are feeling better these days; I am sure that this will be the case. So you know why I am so sure? It is because I went through the same experience with viral encephalitis myself and the same complications, except that my case was more severe.

When I was in Montreal, I heard things about a JAR at the RVH who had a possible deep-seated brain tumor or a possible schizophrenic condition. I knew immediately this case is the same syndrome I had experienced previously. Shall we call it the Forrest-Fox Syndrome?!

At any rate, what I did was to ship up to the Allan and conduct an extensive history of your case while you were still in the amnesic reactive depression phase (I didn't know you were supposed to be under wraps).

This is what I want to do. I don't know how well you are now, but I have had 100 percent recovery and expect to be back in Montreal this summer.

I want you to join with me in writing our experiences with this syndrome associated with viral encephalitis and write it up in a scientific form for the New England Journal of Medicine. You can also assess my case and I'll assess yours. I think it has great possibilities, but this will all depend on how eager you are to do this with me and how well you are. At any rate, I have a full account of the onset and course of the illness should you be amnesic from this stage and wish to see medical notes on it.

I hope this idea fascinates you as it has fascinated me. I shall respond to any request for more details.

Your friend and fellow encephalitic,

Bob Forrest

When I read the letter in 2020, I jumped on Google and, sadly, found his obituary from 2016. Born in Moose Jaw, Saskatchewan, in 1943, he received his MD from the University of Saskatchewan, then came to Montreal for a neurology residency at McGill. The obituary says he caught encephalitis while working at the Montreal Children's Hospital. He must have been severely ill—his recovery was a major battle: "Against all odds, he relearned to speak and walk again, and then went on to relearn his medicine and practiced for many more years in Montreal, Saskatchewan, and British Columbia. Bob was a man of incredible perseverance, tenacity, and resilience, respected by his peers and a mentor to many."

I'm sorry I never got to meet this exceptional man when I was healthy, to hear his story, compare notes, and to find out more about my own illness. From the letter, it sounds as if he was able to gain full access to all my records because he was a doctor in the McGill health system. Looking back, I see that Dr. Forrest and I had some things in common besides our illnesses. We were the same age, both McGill medical residents, and we both took ill within a relatively short time frame with what was probably the same condition. Encephalitis is not all that common of a disease.

Had we connected soon after my discharge, would I have taken him up on his offer to co-author a paper on our illness? Probably not, though it's a tempting idea to contemplate and I feel a twinge of regret. But after discharge, my health status was still uncertain and felt compelled to work hard at the hospital to make up for lost time. And as you'll read in the next chapter, my plate would be heaped sky high for the rest of 1969, with no room for a single additional project.

CHAPTER 10
1969

When my doctors advised a holiday after discharge, followed by a cautious return to work, they were laying out a strategy akin to taxiing on the runway before a smooth takeoff and slow ascent to cruising altitude. Maybe they imagined me stretched out on a lounge chair under a beach umbrella, basking in the beauty of white sands and cerulean waters and breathing in the salty air. A soothing, restorative holiday, calming to mind and body.

Ha! With its ever-changing flow of causes and conditions, life has a way of plotting its own itinerary. To paraphrase poet Robert Burns, the best laid plans of mice and men can go astray.[5] I went home from the AMI on February 19, 1969. Gloria and I heeded the doctors' advice and quickly planned a holiday to Puerto Rico—a popular vacation destination for North Americans. In the cold Canadian winter, a tropical climate and dramatic scenery change seemed like a good way to cleanse the trauma of the last three months. But our Puerto Rico trip fell short of expectations.

Gloria picks up the story: "We must have had a terrible travel agent because we ended up in a US naval base far from the ocean. We were told it was just a fifteen-minute taxi ride, but in fact it was forty-five minutes. We stayed in this hotel,

---

[5.] Robert Burns, "To a Mouse," in *Poems, Chiefly in the Scottish Dialect* (Kilmarnock: John Wilson, 1786), 138–140, https://digital.nls.uk/poems-chiefly-in-the-scottish-dialect/archive/74464614#?c.

and I know we did some side trips. We went to see the rainforest in Puerto Rico." We'd booked the trip on short notice and wound up in a hotel in the middle of nowhere. As to my health, Gloria says it was normal: "Although every time you twitched in bed at night, I was very concerned that it was the start of a seizure." There we were, with me right on the heels of a mysterious illness that might not have been over, stuck in a remote location with the quantity and quality of local medical care unknown. It was a bust.

"We hated being in this place," Gloria adds. "We went to San Juan [the capital] and stayed overnight in a hotel. The planes were flying right over our heads. And we said, 'This is ridiculous! Your [Irving's] grandparents have a lovely house in Saint-Agathe-des-Monts, and perhaps we should just get out of Puerto Rico and go up there.' Which is what we did. Oh, but we had trouble getting back home. There was a snowstorm, so planes were grounded. We finally got a flight into New York." Sainte-Agathe is in the Laurentian Mountains about sixty miles north of Montreal. We went from one airport to another in New York and could not find a flight. "We got onto a bus back to Montreal, went up to Saint-Agathe, and had a lovely few days up there," Gloria recalls. It was a happy time indeed—Gloria became pregnant during our stay.

In hindsight, I wonder if our dissatisfaction with Puerto Rico was less from our accommodations and more from being in an unfamiliar place. I'd spent months in an alien landscape—physically sick with an unknown disease and a psychotic mind, suffering grueling medical tests and bizarre drug side effects. I didn't know if, when, or to what degree I'd recover. Gloria, too, had navigated strange terrain. She was anxious about my health and mental status. Was our future laid to waste? She'd moved in with my parents, which was quite an adjustment, and she had her job teaching seventh graders—something of a feat in itself. After all the chaos, maybe what we craved was not the exotic, but the security of a familiar, comforting environment. A couple of steaming cups of cocoa in front of a roaring fire.

LIFE GOES ON

1969 was a momentous year in the news, with massive cultural and political shifts. Richard Nixon was inaugurated to a US presidency that would end in disgrace in his second term. Protests of the Vietnam War swept across the US, with more than a quarter million people marching peacefully in Washington, DC, in the fall as part of the Moratorium movement to end US involvement.

Beatle John Lennon and his new wife, Yoko Ono, launched their second Bed-In—an eight-day peace promotion—in late May, at the Queen Elizabeth Hotel in Montreal. There, Lennon wrote his antiwar anthem, "Give Peace a Chance," performing it live from the bed in room 1742. (The song was later released by the Plastic Ono Band, not the Beatles.) In August, the Woodstock music festival drew half a million young people to a muddy, rain-drenched farm in upstate New York in what was the counterculture event of the century.

On February 13, I was on the psych ward at AMI. Gloria's father was at another hospital having a leg amputated due to cancer. Needless to say, we weren't focused on the news that afternoon, when the Quebec Liberation Front, an anti-capitalist separatist group, bombed the Montreal Stock Exchange, injuring dozens of people and causing extensive damage to the building.

On July 20, an estimated half billion people watched on TV as astronaut Neil Armstrong became the first man to walk on the moon—an occasion so monumental that it left even the eloquent CBS news anchor, Walter Cronkite, grasping for words. By the late 1960s, the Cold War between the US and the Soviet Union was raging on many fronts, one of which was the Space Race. The Apollo 11 moon landing represented—arguably—a US victory in the Space Race.

Meanwhile, Gloria and I were running a race *from* space and towards normalcy. Thanks to miscues in my brain circuitry, I'd been living in an altered reality that was like visiting another planet. In the first half of 1969, Neil Armstrong (with fellow astronauts Buzz Aldrin and Michael Collins) was preparing for his summer journey to the moon. Me? I felt like I'd just returned from Mars. I'd been on a three-month, spaced-out, outer-space trip and dearly hoped never to go back out there.

Historic, earth-shaking events swirled all around us in 1969. With my illness—we hoped—behind us, Gloria and I wanted to move forward. But our world had been shaken to its roots by my illness. We were relieved and grateful for my near-miraculous recovery, yet we now knew, consciously or not, that no one was exempt from the whims of fate. That knowledge propelled us to always make the most of our lives and our careers of service, and also to start our family.

On a miniature scale, 1969 would be a year as epic in shaping our personal future as all the major news stories were in shaping the global future. I guess it's not surprising that a year that saw me in a psych ward on day one would turn out to be a wild ride all the way through to December. And so it was. After our vacation, I eased back into hospital work. Gloria returned to the classroom. Her father learned to walk with a prosthesis. Then Gloria's aunt was diagnosed with multiple sclerosis.

I had missed a big chunk of my residency and wanted to make up for lost time as best I could. I was slowed down in that effort by my anti-seizure medications, which precluded driving for three months. We were thrilled when we found out Gloria was pregnant, but we barely had time to celebrate while planning our summer move to North Carolina. I was starting the postdoctoral fellowship program at Duke University, in a research training program in the lab of Dr. James Wyngarden, chair of Duke's Department of Medicine.

About a month before we left Canada, Gloria was hospitalized for bleeding and risk of miscarriage. Fortunately, all was well. I flew solo to Halifax, Nova Scotia, to be a groomsman in the wedding of my dear friend Lenny Diamond to Gloria's second cousin. Soon afterwards, we'd leave for Durham, traveling in our prized possession, a 1968 Volvo P1800 coupe with no air conditioning. You can still buy one of these classic cars today. Due to her bleeding, Gloria had to take it easy. "I was unable to pack and sat and watched everybody pack up our small apartment." We shipped seventeen boxes, and two trunks. "And off to Durham we went in our sports car."

DURHAM, NORTH CAROLINA

We left Montreal around July 1. Our possessions arrived in Durham a few days after us and were deposited on the sidewalk in front of our apartment in Duke's married student housing. Some wonderful students came and helped schlep the load up to our third-floor apartment. Our stay in Durham would last three years. Two of our three daughters were born there.

We had much to learn as we embarked on this new stage of our life's adventure together. We had left our roots, our family, and our friends in the Montreal Jewish community. Here we were, expecting a baby, moving to a new home in a city we found very strange and a new research training job for me. Gloria and I surged forward and forgot about my illness. We had a full plate to deal with and no time to look back.

In the present we were in culture shock, not just from being in a new country, but from being in the South. It was just a year after integration. At the Duke hospital, I could see where the lettering over bathrooms reading "Blacks Only" had been incompletely whitewashed. Of course, there was discrimination, racism, and anti-Semitism in Montreal, but neither of us had personally experienced it, nor had we been exposed to the kind of raw hatred of Black people that we saw in North Carolina. Anti-Semitism was also widespread. The bigotry shocked us.

Many of our friends in student housing came from New York, New Jersey, or elsewhere in the Northeast. So we felt a degree of cultural affinity, but it was still difficult. One day, we drove into South Carolina and saw a huge billboard featuring a man in a pointy hat sitting on a rearing horse and holding a cross aloft. It was imagery for United Klans of America, one of the South's most violent Ku Klux Klan organizations. The billboard encouraged people to "Help Fight Communism and Integration."

After our daughter Caroline was born in late 1969, Gloria went back to school, working towards a master's in special education. We were fortunate to hire women from the community, including married student neighbors to take care of Caroline while we were gone.

MESHUGANA MOE AND THE STIGMA

The rapid-fire personal developments of 1969 quickly made ancient history of my illness. At deep levels, I believe our hearts and minds were changed for the better by the ordeal. But we were soon going about our daily activities as if I'd never been ill. We cast the memory aside. Until I started writing this book, I rarely, if ever, revealed to anyone that I'd spent two months in a psychiatric hospital. My condition was a physical illness that caused psychiatric symptoms. However, there was such a huge stigma around mental illness that this was a distinction without a difference. I believed being open about my illness would negatively impact my career and our social circles. We kept mum.

Gloria had been especially worried when I went into the psych hospital. She'd seen how people were stigmatized for mental illness with a relative nicknamed "Meshugana Moe." (Meshugana, meaning crazy person, comes from the

Yiddish.) Moe had a chronic psychiatric disorder, probably schizophrenia. I actually saw him when I was on psychiatric rotation in medical school. The doctors used to trot him out to display his condition to the students. Moe was a sick man, but you can see by the nickname that he was treated like a joke. We wanted to avoid any such stigma.

The bias against mental illness may not be as overt today as it was in the 1960s, but it's still a factor in the medical field, often in subtle ways. In 2021, Dr. Michelle H. Silver wrote a column in the *New England Journal of Medicine* about how she was advised to remove any mention of an eating disorder from her personal statements on medical program applications.[6] It was her own mental illness that motivated her to become a doctor. Yet stating that truth would likely have knocked her out of the running. Dr. Silver notes that due to the nature of the work and the demands of medicine, there's a high level of burnout among medical professionals and trainees that, ironically, leads to higher-than-average rates of mental illnesses such as depression in the field. She feels that the self-censorship and denial actually exacerbate the burnout epidemic.

I'm glad that, now retired, I have the chance to safely discuss my own experience with psychiatric symptoms. But given the circumstances at the time, I think we made the right call to keep it to ourselves.

1969 STARTS IN MISERY, ENDS IN JOY

My daughter Caroline Samara Fox was born on December 1—nine months after my discharge and almost exactly a year since I'd collapsed with a generalized seizure while talking on the phone to Arnie Aberman. Within two weeks of Caroline's birth, I would turn twenty-six and Gloria, twenty-four.

[6.] Michelle H. Silver, "The Good Fit—Why Medical Applicants' Personal Statements Are Anything but Personal," *New England Journal of Medicine* 384, no. 12 (March 25, 2021): 1086–1087, https://doi.org/10.1056/NEJMp2032383.

Was it youthful recklessness for us to get pregnant so soon after my illness? Maybe. But never, even for a second, have we regretted the decision.

In my personal notes from the first part of my illness, I feared having a fatal brain tumor and felt drawn to the idea of having a child. Gloria says the baby was my way of leaving something behind. She says, "Of course I was nervous because I had no idea what was going to happen. I became pregnant not knowing what Irving's prognosis was." I might have left Gloria as a young widow, raising a baby on her own. Thank goodness this was a risk that paid off handsomely!

Despite her hesitation, Gloria says that deep down she always believed I'd get better. And once my recovery did get underway, everything happened so fast: "I had a concern, but it was very fleeting. I was dealing with moment to moment to moment. Boom, you're better and life became normal again. Boom, we were traveling to North Carolina and settling in there."

After all we'd gone through that year, you'd think karma might smile on our first childbirth, but it didn't—at least not initially. Caroline spent her first two weeks in the neonatal intensive care unit after being born in fetal distress. As you can imagine, this put Gloria and me in parental distress. Gloria recalls expressing her concerns to one particularly callous resident: "I asked the resident, 'Is she really sick? Is she going to die?' He answered, "Well, babies aren't in here for their health, you know. They're all sick.'" Not exactly a paradigm of compassion, was he?

It all worked out just fine. Caroline came home from the intensive care unit and was a very healthy baby who brought us endless joy. She would become a big sister in a little more than a year, while we were still living in Durham.

CHAPTER 11
Recovery and the Gift of Life

Chanukah and Christmas came and went in 1969, wrapping up the year with a monster Christmas nor'easter that brought record snowfall to Montreal and killed fifteen people throughout Quebec. Of course, it can freeze or snow in Durham, but compared to what we were used to in Canada, the North Carolina winter felt positively balmy. New Year's Eve brought a little storm to Durham, with four inches of snow. We'd been invited to a party and found ourselves the only guests. Durham residents were so put off by the snow that they all stayed home.

We had our first American Thanksgiving in late November that year. (Canada observes the holiday in October.) Four days later, we really had something to be thankful for, as our little branch of the Fox family grew to three with the birth of our daughter Caroline. I spent my twenty-fifth birthday in the hospital on December 7, 1968. What a bizarre twist that my next birthday would see my week-old baby girl hospitalized, recovering from fetal distress. Happily, she was home with us by Gloria's birthday a week later and suffered no lingering effects.

What a year! Baby Caroline and I had both faced potentially life-threatening conditions. Gloria confronted a threat of miscarriage during her pregnancy, plus serious illnesses of close family members. I missed three months of my medical training, but somehow managed to complete it and land a postdoctoral fellowship that necessitated moving to the US with my pregnant wife, both of us struggling with culture shock as we adjusted to life in the American South.

How on God's green earth did we manage to keep on keepin' on—and do so at such a high level of intensity? Looking back, I think much of it was due to our raw, youthful exuberance and the drive to keep pursuing our goals and dreams. Gloria and I were raised with confidence and self-worth. When adversity struck, as it did repeatedly that year, we didn't wallow in self-pity. Yes, we were scared. Who wouldn't be? But we were undaunted. We acted as if things would work out, and they did. We kept calm and carried on.

My miraculous recovery the previous February was the gift of a lifetime for us in more ways than one. I not only improved but recovered fully, with no brain damage, ongoing seizures, or other lasting effects. It was a gift that all my time off didn't derail me from the trajectory of my medical career. There were also subtle gifts tucked inside the bigger package, such as lessons we learned and later applied, often without even knowing it. We did the best we could, gaining resilience that enabled us to cope next time a curve ball was thrown. We bore the weight of our burdens without whining, developing strength and stamina as a result. Our tolerance for risk increased. Our compassion and empathy grew.

We learned that in all its fragility, life itself is a gift to cherish. The hardships we endured bolstered our values and commitments to family, friends, education, and service. We both chose work in which we could make contributions to society, and we promoted similar values in our children. With the gift of recovery, we embarked on a life adventure that always kept us grounded, even when short-term positive outcomes weren't assured. I'm going to walk you through some of the highlights of my personal and family life, and in the next chapter we'll explore my career achievements, including patient care, research, and drug development that dramatically improved the quality of life of hundreds of thousands of people.

PROCREATION: HARD WORK, BUT SOMEONE'S GOTTA DO IT

I was the oldest of three kids in a family of five. Gloria, however, was the only child in her natal family. She was bound and determined for us to have more than one child. It was with a single-minded focus that Gloria was, shall we say, quite proactive about achieving that goal. Procreation can be fun, though I admit it was often exhausting after my long hours at work. But our efforts paid off beautifully when we welcomed Sharon Lee Fox to the family on January 17, 1971, in Durham—thirteen months after her big sister Caroline. With my work, Gloria's school, limited earnings, and now two kids in diapers, our plates were fuller than ever. But we were thrilled with our two girls. No complaints, no regrets.

Education was a core value. We loved learning! After Caroline's birth, Gloria enrolled at the University of North Carolina at Chapel Hill, earning her master's degree in special education in 1972. She might have started school earlier, but she waited until we'd been state residents for six months in order to qualify for reduced in-state tuition. That was necessary because our income from my fellowship stipend was extremely limited. Dr. Wyngaarden, Chair of Duke's Department of Medicine and head of the lab where I was learning research, determined that my income was below the poverty level. Dr. Wyngaarden helped ease the burden by generously arranging a supplement to my stipend. That gave us a little breathing room.

At Duke, I was a postdoctoral fellow for two years, then a senior resident in medicine for a third. My fellowship mentor was Dr. William N. Kelley, a man of extraordinary skill, talent, expertise, and leadership ability who taught me a tremendous amount.[7] He became a good friend and would play another key role in my career at a later stage of my life. We made important discoveries at the research bench in the lab and clinical studies with patients, publishing significant articles in prominent medical journals. Bill Kelley ultimately became quite famous in academic medicine, going on to become Chair of Medicine at the University of Michigan (U-M) and CEO/Dean at Penn Medicine at the University of Pennsylvania.

BACK TO THE LAND OF THE MAPLE LEAF

In 1972, Gloria received her master's in special education, and that June I completed my rheumatology fellowship and senior residency in medicine at Duke University. This was another turning point for us. I was honored to be offered two different faculty jobs at Duke's School of Medicine—in rheumatology and cardiology. We had two children younger than three, lived in a very different kind of culture, and were far from family. We wanted to return to Canada. Another factor was the US draft. The bloody Vietnam War was still raging

---

7. EW Holmes, Of rice and men: Bill Kelley's next generation. J Clin Invest 2005; 115, 2948-2952

in 1972. At twenty-seven and being a US resident, I would be eligible to be drafted as a physician until age thirty-five.

I accepted a position in Toronto after receiving many offers from medical schools across Canada. I was appointed Assistant Professor of Medicine at the University of Toronto, located at the university-affiliated Wellesley Hospital, part of the Rheumatic Diseases Unit. This is where I started my laboratory devoted to purine metabolism and gout and also my small private rheumatology practice.

Rheumatic diseases are autoimmune or inflammatory diseases that affect the musculoskeletal system—the joints, bones, tendons, and other structures that allow the body to move. Osteoarthritis is probably the most well-known of these, which also include rheumatoid arthritis, gout, scleroderma, psoriatic arthritis, lupus, and fibromyalgia, among many, many others. We'll delve more into this subject when we discuss my career in the next chapter.

We lived in Toronto from 1972 until 1976. Gloria worked as a special education teacher, and our two girls developed through toddlerhood. Caroline started school in Toronto. We had a good life there, buying a home and making friends. My sister Rosanne and her husband, Steve, lived in Toronto, so we had family ties. We saw them frequently. The only odd thing was that professionally we were made to feel like outsiders. I don't know why; perhaps because we're not originally from Toronto. Otherwise, my experience at the University of Toronto was productive and fun. Thanks to successful grant applications, my lab was well-funded and our team did substantive work that was published in a variety of important medical and scientific journals.

My friend and wonderful Duke mentor, Dr. Bill Kelley became Chair of the Department of Internal Medicine (usually just called "Medicine") at the University of Michigan (U-M) Medical School in Ann Arbor in 1975. At the tender age of thirty-six, he was young to hold such a post and, in fact, was the youngest such chair in the US. I accepted his offer to join him there in 1976—the first of what would become more than 150 recruits who would come to Michigan and help Bill Kelley transform the department to one of the foremost in the country.

My term at the University of Toronto Medical School ended on a slightly sour personal note for me. This was unrelated to the university and occurred through no fault of theirs. When I announced my plans to move to Ann Arbor, I was used as a pawn to sensationalize a difficult period of medical research funding in Canada. Without permission, the *Toronto Star* newspaper printed a page 2 photo of me holding a test tube over the caption "Researcher heads south to escape financial freeze." My lab actually had excellent funding, and the headline was simply untrue. This was personally upsetting, especially when my letter to the editor to correct the record was buried in an obscure part of a subsequent edition.

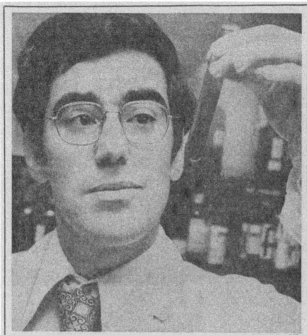

ARTHRITIS RESEARCHER Dr. Irving Fox of Wellesley Hospital is leaving Toronto July 1 for a post at the University of Michigan largely because of the cut in federal support for medical research in Canada. He is "one of the brightest young medical scientists in the country," a top doctor says.

Researcher is heading south to escape the financial freeze

By MARILYN DUNLOP
Star staff writer

The University of Toronto is losing "one of the brightest young medical scientists in the country" largely because of inadequate federal government support for medical research, a top Toronto doctor said yesterday.

Dr. Charles Hollenberg, chief of the U of T's department of medicine, disclosed that Dr. Irving Fox, an arthritis researcher at Wellesley Hospital, will leave Toronto July 1 to take a post at the University of Michigan.

"I regard his loss as a most serious loss in the department of medicine," Hollenberg said.

Hollenberg cited the loss as an example of damage to medicine in Canada that will result from a freeze put on the Medical Research Council's budget by the federal government.

The council, a government agency, assesses research and distributes more than half the $80 million spent on medical research in Canada.

Its budget this year is set at $43.5 million, no more than it got last year despite inflation, which, scientists say, has increased the cost of research 15 per cent.

Commenting on the freeze, Hollenberg said angrily: "This is the most unwise thing the federal government has done. I am a life-long Liberal. But I must say it—this is the most damaging thing I've seen done."

He said the government is denying talented Canadians the opportunity "to fulfill themselves within Canada. They will do it someplace. Why not in Canada?"

Fox, he said, is a brilliant Canadian: "We've done our damndest to keep him.

"But we just can't match the opportunity he's been offered. People of that quality can command the best in equipment and opportunity. There were undoubtedly other factors that led to his decision but certainly, the uncertainty of government funding played a role."

Fox, who will become director of clinical research at the University of Michigan, said in an interview he decided to leave because the opportunity to expand his research was much greater in the U.S.

"It was a difficult decision," he said, "You do not make such a decision lightly. I will be only 40 miles from the border but it is not the same as being in Canada."

Fox, born and educated in Montreal, took postgraduate training at Duke University in North Carolina and returned to Toronto in 1972.

Funds for his research into arthritis and gout came from three sources — the Medical Research Council, the Arthritis Society and the Ontario Heart Foundation for a total of more than $80,000. Most of that pays salaries of technicians in his laboratory.

Of the total, the Medical Research Council provided $22,000 last year and promised to increase his grant by $2,000 this year. However the freeze forced the council to cut back three per cent ($720).

Fox said he did not want to give the impression his leaving was "sour grapes." "I can't complain about my treatment in Canada."

● Scientists are alarmed at the freeze on medical research funds. But researchers at Toronto's Wellesley Hospital are making breakthroughs in medicine. Details, page B3.

This picture and article were published in the Toronto Star in 1976.
From Toronto Star. © [publication 1976 of Licensed Content] Toronto Star Newspapers Limited. All rights reserved. Used under license.

STATESIDE: ANN ARBOR, MICHIGAN

If you hop into your car in Toronto and head southwest, above the North Shore of Lake Erie, you can be at the U-M in less than five hours. Our move ought to have been smooth sailing. It wasn't. I guess that's not surprising, given the intensely active pace of our lives back then. Gloria once again found herself relocating while pregnant—this time with two very young children in tow. At the end of June 1976, she was just about halfway through her third pregnancy.

Before moving, we had been to a medical conference in Europe, cutting it close by coming back to Toronto only three days before our scheduled move on July 1. Just as we arrived home, my H1 visa was delivered. This was a temporary work visa granted to foreigners in certain employment categories that were highly sought-after in the US. Without it, I couldn't have worked in the US. We had sold our house in Toronto and were already building a new one in Ann Arbor, but it wouldn't be ready for another two or three months. So we had to rent, which meant we'd get settled in for the summer and then have to pack up yet again when our new house was ready—a move that would happen during Gloria's third trimester.

Honestly! Now that we're retired and our life is largely tamed by COVID-19, I can't imagine taking the risk of tossing all those balls into the air without a clue as to where and how they might land. Were we naive? You bet! But consider this: Seven years earlier, we didn't know if I would live, die, or be permanently disabled. I didn't know my left foot from my right. I'd told my friend Arnie that a doctor brought me down to the hospital basement to pray to his dead mother in a coffin. I told Gloria I'd been speaking to my friend Lenny through a tube in a hospital wall. By 1976, we never thought about my illness, but we knew how to cope and do what we had to do. We were young, dauntless, and bold.

Once we got settled, things worked out quite favorably in Ann Arbor. My academic appointments at the U-M included both Associate Professor of Internal Medicine and Assistant Professor of Biological Chemistry. I also had an appointment as Associate Director of the Clinical Research Center, and I became Director a year later. My research lab was set up in the Clinical Research Center.

My H1 visa allowed me to work in the US for up to four years. Gloria didn't have one, so she couldn't work. This was fine at first, with Joanna born soon after our move and Gloria's hands full. Then, in 1977, the US announced that due to a shortage of physicians, people like me would be given priority to apply for permanent residency—a green card. Soon Gloria and I officially became permanent residents with most of the privileges of US citizenship, except for voting. The green card was a green light for Gloria to find a job, which she eventually did.

We lived happily in Ann Arbor for about fourteen years. Our youngest child, Joanna Lynn Fox, was born on November 16, 1976, at the U-M Medical Center. People were critical of us having a third child. In 1976, the concept of zero population growth was quite the rage in Ann Arbor! All the girls went to local public schools. We lived on Andover Street, just off U-M's north campus. With about forty thousand students and people from all over the country and the world, our girls were exposed to a diversity of people and experiences.

Gloria and I were philosophically in sync about child-rearing. We encouraged our daughters to pursue any careers they wished and to ignore the historical, gender-based stereotypes and biases. We were committed to helping them discover and follow their own dreams. Caroline once complained to me that the world was not fair to women. I agreed and told her she'd have to pursue excellence and attain career positions in which she could help change gender injustice. All our daughters earned their college undergraduate degrees at U-M, which consistently ranks among the top universities in the country. Caroline was an English major and pre-med, later receiving a master's in public health. Both Sharon and Joanna had the same major—industrial and operations engineering.

Gloria and I found life in Ann Arbor to be very fulfilling as we became part of the friendly and engaging community. We joined Temple Beth Emeth, where I was elected vice president and then president. I also became President of the Genesis Board, which oversaw the synagogue's shared building with St. Clare's Episcopal Church. This unique union of Jewish and Episcopal houses of worship gained national publicity when it was established in 1976. The location is marked by the cross and the Star of David standing together in the front of the building.

Gloria earned another diploma, this one in instructional technology. She became a teacher at the Solomon Schechter School, a private network of day schools in the conservative Jewish tradition. Gloria taught a combined class of third-, fourth-, and fifth-grade students. She didn't work there long, however, because we decided to leave Ann Arbor and relocate once more.

It was December 1989, a month after Joanna's bat mitzvah, when I made the very difficult decision together with Gloria to leave academic medicine and join the biotechnology industry, which was in its early stages and growing rapidly. I did plenty of soul searching, taking a long, hard look at my career progress up to that time. Asking myself how much I had changed patient treatment with my research work, I candidly answered, "not substantially." I felt that the metric for success in the biotech pharmaceutical industry was developing effective new medicines. Since improving treatments was one of my key career goals, biotech was the place for me to be.

I got plenty of flak from some of my colleagues, who urged me not to toss my academic medicine career out the window. One said, "You're the ultimate academic. I cannot imagine you working in industry." Another felt I wasn't cut out for it: "How will you deal with those sleazeball businessmen?" These were colleagues I liked and respected. There was some merit in their thinking that excessive greed and the profit motive can have poisonous effects on the human spirit. But my heart told me to go where I could do the work that meant the most to me with my usual high level of scientific rigor and integrity. And that's what happened.

Another factor was at play that made the decision a little easier. In 1989, only about 10 or 15 percent of individual approved grants at the National Institutes of Health were actually being funded. The lack of adequate government funding was forcing me to spend a growing chunk of my time writing grants to gain support for my research lab. That was a low cost-benefit ratio for my time and effort. I wanted to find new treatments to help people who were suffering, not to increase my own suffering by constantly going hat in hand looking for money. That settled things. Sadly, it was "bye-bye" to Ann Arbor and a community we had come to love.

THE BIGGEST RISK YET

The move from Ann Arbor wasn't like the others. I was forty-six when I made the big leap into biotech, an age when many doctors have put down strong roots in established careers and communities. I accepted an offer from Biogen in Cambridge, Massachusetts, having been recruited by Jim Vincent, the CEO. Jim was quite the salesman. He called me at midnight in December 1989, when Gloria and I were in bed, and talked about the "Wallenda" principal to seal the deal. It was emblematic of the change I was making that my new boss had a background in engineering and business, not medicine. My title at Biogen was Vice President of Clinical Research.

Compared to academic medicine, this was a whole new world of business recruitment, with forgivable loans, base salary, bonus and stock options, and a severance agreement. Processes and procedures were radically different from those I knew. Dress for senior executives in the early 1990s was more formal than for academics. My leather knapsack and Clarks Wallabees were quickly exchanged for "big boy shoes" (wingtips and cap toes), suits with vests, and a briefcase.

Job tenure in business was based on level of performance each year. My generous financial package made our family whole for a home purchase in the Boston area, where prices were double those of Ann Arbor in 1990. Nevertheless, my contract was such that I faced financial ruin if I quit or got fired during my first two years at Biogen. If I left before two years, I would have to return the money. Gulp!

Academic medicine and research weren't the most lucrative fields at the time, and I had plenty of debt. I had two kids enrolled at U-M, not exactly a low-cost ticket. I'd put everything at risk with this shift into what was truly unknown. There was no going back. I would sink or swim based upon my own performance, personal ability, skills, and resilience. In the end, I swam. After several years, I led my team to achieve approval of Avonex, a treatment for multiple sclerosis.

It took until my mid-forties to look in the mirror and see who I was: a risk taker. Drug development is for risk takers.

Who else would cheerfully embark on a task in which the chance of achieving a drug approval was one in ten? In 1990, for every ten drugs in clinical research, only one would emerge from the pipeline and gain marketing authorization.

I rented a flat in Back Bay in Boston and began work at Biogen on February 1, 1990. Gloria and Joanna would join me about a month later, when we moved to a townhouse in Wellesley, in suburban Boston. At thirteen and in her last half-year of middle school, Joanna was traumatized by the move, as she had started at a middle school in Wellesley where she knew no one and all the courses were different. After six weeks, she desperately wanted to return to her friends and school in Ann Arbor. We had followed the advice of guidance counselors to move her sooner rather than later so that she'd have time to adjust before starting a new high school. Joanna struggled through and, resilient girl that she was, adjusted, but it wasn't until the next school year. Gloria and I thought we could've found a better way to help her with a difficult transition into which she'd had no input.

Joanna wasn't the only one needing time to adjust. Gloria and I found Wellesley markedly different from Ann Arbor, where, due to the university, just about everyone came from somewhere else and newcomers were quickly embraced. But bonds in Wellesley seemed to develop more slowly and tentatively. We were used to often getting together with friends and family who lived close to us. In the Boston area, that wasn't the case. People seemed more socially aloof. When the telephone rang, it was either the wrong number or a long-distance call.

We needed to find a different way to make friends and connect in the community. We did that by joining a local synagogue, Temple Beth Elohim. And Gloria became a gallery instructor at the Museum of Fine Arts in Boston. This created an environment where Gloria could do what she loves so dearly: learning and teaching. And it also offered opportunities for meeting new people and making new friends. As part of her volunteer work, Gloria led school children on tours of the museum. The museum affiliation was so wonderful that it continues to be an important part of Gloria's life today and has fostered many of our enduring friendships as a couple.

In 1992, Gloria and I were pleased to become naturalized American citizens. We were a bit weary of having taxation without representation—being unable to vote for those representing us. Now we could fully participate in American democracy. Our children had dual American and Canadian citizenship. Meanwhile, our older daughters were at first reluctant to join us in Wellesley since all their friends were in Ann Arbor. But they did come eventually. At first it took bribery such as, "If you come home this weekend, Mommy will take you shopping." Eventually, they saw the light and moved to Boston for longer periods and life-changing opportunities.

FAMILY MATTERS

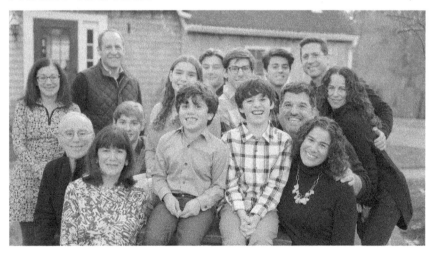

This Fox Family photograph was taken on Thanksgiving in 2022. This photograph was taken by the author's grandson, Jamie Spielman.

Caroline graduated med school at the University of Pennsylvania and was accepted for her house officer training at Boston's Brigham and Women's Hospital. She met Dr. Steve Wiviott when they were both on call at the hospital. They married in 2001, settling near us in Boston, both with academic positions at Harvard Medical School. Caroline attained a professorship at Harvard and tenure at the National Institutes of Health with the Framingham Heart Study. She left those positions in 2015 for a job as Vice President at Merck Research Labs in Boston. Steve was honored by being promoted to full Professor of Medicine at Harvard Medical School and is a vice president at Mass General Brigham. They have three teenagers.

Sharon worked in consulting in New York for a couple of years, then attended Harvard Business School, where she met Matt Spielman, her future husband. They moved to New York, married in 2000, and now live in Scarsdale, New York, with two teenage sons. Sharon is a private equity operating partner and sits on the boards of public and portfolio companies. Matt runs a successful executive coaching business. He has some celebrity clients and has appeared as a guest on *Good Morning America*. Matt's recent book about executive coaching, titled *Inflection Points*, has gained substantial recognition upon publication in 2022.

After a rough start, Joanna graduated Wellesley High in 1996, then attended U-M in the industrial and operational engineering program. She worked in telecommunications for Sprint in Kansas City, then moved back to Wellesley and joined a telecommunications startup that went belly up. She then enrolled at Penn, earned a master's in math education, and taught high school math in Boston. She got a second master's at Harvard so she could become a school principal. She met Jonathan Wasserman when he was a doctor in training at Harvard Children's Hospital. They married in 2008 and moved to Jonathan's hometown of Toronto. Jonathan works at the Hospital for Sick Children and is associate professor at the University of Toronto. Joanna is a principal of a school for kindergarten to eighth grade. They have two sons.

Family is of paramount importance to Gloria and me, and we've created rituals that strengthen our bonds. We've produced the annual "Fox Family Newsletter" every December for more than twenty-five years. We gather with family as often as we can on Jewish holidays and other occasions, and we go on a family vacation each December when the grandkids are off school. Most of this has been stymied by the pandemic. During vacations, the adults hold a family meeting to discuss everything from family interactions to our wills and investment portfolios. Some of our older grandsons have started clamoring to attend these meetings.

Our three daughters produced a passel of boys. We have six grandsons and one granddaughter. All of them—daughters, sons-in-law, and grandchildren—fill us with joy. As I write this, Gloria and I have been happily married for fifty-six years. We marked our milestone golden anniversary in June 2016 with a major bash for family and friends. Two months later, our celebration continued with a family trip to Alaska. We recognize how fortunate we are to have had such a great life, an enduring marriage, and an extraordinary family, and we celebrate each day as the gift that it is.

CHAPTER 12
Risky Business

In the Irving Fox Operations Manual, you won't find instructions for dipping a cautious toe in the chilly water and gradually getting wet. There's no setting for incremental. Oh, I plan, analyze, consult with my wife, and think things through. But once I make up my mind, I tend to plunge right in—maybe not quite as gracefully as those cliff divers Gloria and I watched on our long-ago vacation in Acapulco.

I was alone in a new apartment in a new city, with a new and unfamiliar job in a burgeoning new industry, with an operational structure that was entirely new to me. I had a new boss whose management style was unlike that of anyone I'd known, and my new contract had a do-or-die clause that put me at a new level of financial risk. There was no gentle transition. I moved into my Back Bay, Boston apartment on January 31, 1990, woke up the next day, donned a suit and tie, and made my way to my new office at Biogen in Cambridge.

I barely had time to hang up my coat and shake a few hands before CEO Jim Vincent called the new vice president of clinical research into his office. I was used to dealing with doctors, but Jim, a Wharton MBA, was a different breed: a large, imposing man with a brusque, army-general leadership style. He got right to the point. Biogen was pouring 20 percent of its budget into a soluble CD4 drug to treat HIV infection, with two clinical trials that had no patients.

"What," he demanded, "are you going to do about this?" I left his office with that echoing in my head: "Shit! What am I going to do about this?" I would shut down the product in less than a year, after determining it was fatally flawed. But that meeting was the beginning of my biotech baptism by fire.

Throwing caution to the wind, I had leaped into a new world I didn't understand. This was the biggest risk I'd ever taken, but it wasn't the first time I found myself in such a pickle. When I began my career at the University of Toronto in 1972, I became involved in rheumatology, an emerging medical specialty. The minimal amount of time I'd spent treating arthritis patients at Duke was the extent of my clinical experience with rheumatic diseases—almost none. In fact, I learned clinical rheumatology on the job at the university's Wellesley Hospital, thanks to my clinically competent and incredibly patient colleague, the late Dr. Hugh Smyth.

Now here I was again, my future hinged on my ability to learn on my feet. When it came to patience, Jim Vincent was no Hugh Smyth. My early years at Biogen were a rough ride, partly because of my steep learning curve, but also because Vincent was not easy to get along with. Frankly, we were like oil and water. On management retreats to Vermont, he'd play poker and smoke cigars into the wee hours. I'd turn in early, then go for a morning bike ride through the Vermont hills.

To his credit, Vincent pulled off a turnaround that most thought impossible. Like many biotech firms back then, Biogen was bleeding money, spending lavishly on research and development (R&D) as well as on salaries. Since no drugs had reached the market, no black ink appeared on the balance sheet. Vincent trimmed fat, reduced staff, streamlined processes, and honed the company's focus. I benefitted from his mentoring, as brutal as it often was. I wasn't the only one who found it rough. When I began, there were thirteen of us on the senior management team. Four years later, only three remained: the CEO, the head of human resources, and me. The rest had quit or been fired, and one died tragically by suicide.

In my new role, I found that getting a new drug to market was much harder than I ever imagined. We had clinical trials in dozens of locations worldwide, dealing with all kinds of local sociopolitical issues while maintaining the high standards of science and tackling all the regulatory processes in each country. A high performing multidisciplinary team with strong leadership is essential for success since no person can do this alone. Building a team to execute studies and shuttle a drug to the finish line meant constant problem-solving. In my own learning process, I developed four axioms of clinical drug development:

1. **Time is a consumable, non-renewable resource.** Once lost, it cannot be recovered.

2. **In drug development, the exception is the rule.** There are so many unique problems to solve every day that they become routine, almost humdrum.

3. **Do it right, do it once.** A CEO I knew once noted that no one seems to have time to do things right the first time, then they have to make time to do the tasks again.

4. **Work with speed and quality.** Timelines and deliverables are corporate buzzwords, with supervisors always pressing for faster production, unaware that speed and quality are a pair. There's truth in the old adage, "The perfect is the enemy of the good," yet we also say, "Haste makes waste." The key to success is creating a system that supports speed and quality simultaneously.

BLOCKBUSTER BREAKTHROUGH
AND A DREAM FULFILLED

Those first years at Biogen were grueling, stressful, and frustrating. After the sink-or-swim clause of my contract expired, I could have thrown in the towel and found another job. Instead, I hung in through this intense, boot-camp experience. I learned to push back against the demands of my boss, Jim Vincent, saying to myself, "The worst you can do is fire me, and I can always find another job."

What kept me going? I was fueled by my core personal mission: improving the effectiveness of treatments available to sick people. I wanted to reduce suffering, and I wasn't about to let a little hard work or corporate dysfunction stand in my way. I'd been through the wringer before. Back in Ann Arbor, I took over for a couple of years as interim division chief in rheumatology, keeping my other roles. I worked impossibly long hours, slept four hours a night, and barely saw my family.

The drive to develop new treatments led me to intentionally make drug approval and marketing authorization my personal criteria for success. My passion was to develop and gain approval for novel products that could change paradigms and profoundly improve patient treatment using biotechnology methods and cutting-edge science. Success with a single unique drug could improve the lives of hundreds of thousands of people. I never lost sight of that goal, which is why I was willing to assume huge challenges and tremendous personal risks.

A great drug that meets an important medical need in a new way is a superb commercial opportunity. It generates a healthy flow of revenue to support operations and bring a return on investment (ROI) to shareholders. When a new medicine generates more than a billion dollars a year in sales, it's known as a blockbuster drug, which is a rare occurrence. I worked on many drugs at Biogen and was privileged to lead a fantastic team that won approval for a blockbuster that satisfied my goal of helping large numbers of people and transformed Biogen into a profitable independent company and a major player in the biopharmaceutical industry.

The drug is Avonex, a biopharmaceutical, or biologic, used to treat multiple sclerosis. Avonex was approved in the US in 1996, in the European Union in 1997, and in numerous other countries in 1998 and beyond. With Avonex, patients with multiple sclerosis had a unique new medicine that was the first to definitively show it could slow the progression of disability from this autoimmune disease. Avonex was a tremendous breakthrough in the treatment of multiple sclerosis and a milestone advance in the biotech industry.

I had hired extraordinarily talented people who were key to the success of Avonex and Biogen's continued excellence in drug development. One of my personal coaches once asked me, "Aren't you worried all your direct reports want your job?" "Not at all," I replied. "I only get worried if they can't do their jobs." A test of a strong leader is whether their team thrives after they leave. That's what happened when I departed Biogen in early 1999. I had developed my own effective management skills and quiet leadership style that empowered others to do their best work. For this, I credited Jim Vincent's brutal mentoring, personal coaching, my increasing self-awareness, and valuable anonymous feedback from my team members.

My successes at Biogen spurred me to start my own product development consulting business that was focused on clinical drug development. Most of the consulting I did was with Millennium Pharmaceuticals, a Cambridge-based biopharma firm that was founded in 1993. By the fall of 1999, I became an employee at Millennium, serving initially as sort of an executive utility infielder for this very young company and contributing at the levels of systems and structures, processes, and products. I worked in various capacities with teams developing treatments for leukemia, multiple myeloma, and inflammatory bowel disease.

In 2005, Millennium gave me the title of Distinguished Medical Fellow of Clinical Development, and the following year I was appointed head of inflammation clinical research. Millennium was acquired in 2008 by Takeda Pharmaceuticals, a huge, multinational company based in Osaka, Japan, that was founded more than 240 years ago. I was thrilled to lead the clinical team that achieved the 2014 approval of the breakthrough drug Entyvio, used in the treatment of ulcerative colitis and Crohn's disease. With a unique mechanism of action, Entyvio was safer and more effective than previous drugs used to treat these very difficult diseases. Entyvio gained approval and marketing authorization in 2014 and quickly became a blockbuster. Its TV ads are a potent reminder of the important contribution of our development team.

I retired from Takeda at the end of 2018, but not before taking on an exciting project in my last five years: running an R&D leadership academy intended to "enhance the quality of thought of senior R&D leaders" at the request of the late Tachi Yamada, the head of R&D. Another new challenge, and once again, I set out seeking to learn. My daughter Sharon recommended some leadership training books, which gave me a few ideas. With several Takeda colleagues assisting, we established a collaboration with MIT's Sloan School of Management and developed a unique curriculum, operational plan, and budget.

The leadership academy launched with forty senior Takeda R&D executives from four continents, meeting at MIT in Cambridge. I also offered voluntary confidential individual mentoring. It was a challenge given the participants' broad diversity, but what an incredible educational opportunity—for me as well as my mentees! The academy was a great success, running for three years. I learned that, harnessed effectively, diversity can give a company a competitive edge by enhancing the creativity of teams tasked with critical projects.

ACADEMIC MEDICINE AND A SURPRISE DIAGNOSIS

The thing about full plates is that even when they're heaped high, you can find room for another tasty morsel. Working in academic medicine had long been a part of my constitution. So, from 1991 until 2008, I made room in my exacting schedule for a part-time role as Clinical Professor of Medicine at Harvard Medical School, with appointments for nine years at Massachusetts General Hospital (MGH) and then eight years at Beth Israel Deaconess Medical Center (BIDMC).

I lectured in biochemistry at Harvard and consulted at the MGH Arthritis Clinic, where I taught and supervised trainees in general medicine and rheumatology. I sat on the Advisory Committee of the Clinical Investigator Training Program, which was a joint program of Harvard and MIT. I lectured on clinical drug development in a graduate program at MIT. At BIDMC, I was a member of the rheumatology division, joined the hospital's Board of Trustees in 2003, and then was appointed Trustee Emeritus in 2009.

An unhappy and ironic twist occurred when I was switching appointments from MGH to BIDMC in 1999. Tests I took as part of a health service exam revealed I lacked immunity to rubella, also known as German measles. I guess I never developed immunity from catching it as a child, before the vaccine existed. Rubella is usually a mild disease in childhood but can be quite serious in adults, especially among pregnant women. It can cause fetal mortality or lifelong problems when the child is born. I got the vaccine to protect myself and hospital patients. Four weeks later, I developed inflammatory polyarthritis, meaning inflammation in multiple joints at the same time. That diagnosis evolved into rheumatoid arthritis, a chronic autoimmune disease in the category of my own medical specialty area, rheumatology.

More than twenty years later, my rheumatoid arthritis has been ably managed to remission by a brilliant physician scientist, Dr. Michael Weinblatt, at Brigham and Women's Hospital. My illness a half century ago increased my compassion as a doctor treating patients and as a scientist working respectfully with study subjects. Now my personal experience with rheumatoid arthritis has enhanced my empathy for the arthritis patients under my care. Every cloud has a silver lining.

My ability to show empathy to clinical study subjects in Toronto and Ann Arbor highlights one of the differences between an academic medical environment and the private-sector pharmaceutical business. My university research studies were grant-funded and usually fairly small. I was able to develop a rapport with each participant, thoroughly explaining what the research could and could not do for them and making sure they understood the risks. In the industry—for good reason—such intimate connections weren't possible. There's no way to relate individually to thousands of people enrolled in the trials. Instead, I would try to develop a rapport with the doctors and nurses at each trial site, but even that was tricky. With Entyvio, for example, we had about four hundred sites in thirty-nine countries where sixty different languages were spoken. Companies like Takeda could easily drop $500 million on a late-stage global study, creating enormous pressure for those managing and executing the research. There's no time to sit down face to face with an elderly gout patient hoping to help medical science bring better treatments to the table in her grandchildren's time.

I could spend many pages comparing academic medicine with corporate drug development. But the point isn't to stack them up against each other, because one is not better than the other. Both are important, necessary, and intertwined in the functions they serve in society. Working in both fields brought me the satisfaction of fulfilling key professional goals. I didn't leave my full-time career in academic medicine because I was unhappy. To the contrary, I loved being in the university medical environment where I could flourish in that wonderful mixture of learning, teaching, treating patients, and discovering.

It's true I usually spend time securing grants to pursue specific areas of research interest and satisfy my scientific curiosity. But I found joy in performing basic and clinical research to expand scientific knowledge that might delineate the cause and treatment of human disease. I demonstrated tangible accomplishments in publishing my research in prestigious journals, which helped in obtaining ongoing funding for my research. I was equally pleased about the students, postdoctoral fellows, and faculty members whom I had mentored and influenced over the years.

I left academic medicine and entered the second phase of my career in biotech drug development to pursue my goal of improving patient care by shepherding new treatments from bench to bedside. At first, I found myself stunned as I moved from a world where research, ideas, education, and scientific methods were idealized into a corporate world where creating a product requires enormous numbers of people as well as expense and complexity. It takes a village to perform basic research, conduct animal safety studies, and invent the drug. Pharmaceutical companies must then follow highly regulated processes to manufacture the drug to scale and execute clinical trials. Global clinical studies for successful drug approvals, especially in the late stages, require excellent operational execution along with strict regulatory compliance and creative rigorous scientific work.

If the drug is safe and effective, the manufacturer must then obtain marketing authorization from different regulatory agencies worldwide in order to market and sell the drug. Although most people associate great profits with Big Pharma, the money doesn't necessarily come easily. Drugs fail in clinical studies far more often than they succeed. Part of the expense of drug development is paying for studies of drugs that fail, not just for those that go to market.

One way to consider the complexity of drug development is to think about the stakeholders who must be satisfied by the results of a clinical development program for a new medicine. These stakeholders include sick patients, doctors in practice and in academic medicine, regulatory agencies overseeing the studies, investors in the company, third-party payors, and the corporate executives in charge of running the company.

Talk about culture shock! How was a physician scientist like me supposed to segue from a public university to a complex system with great interest in the bottom line? As a drug developer, I regarded great sales results as our "applause," a sign that people are buying the drug because they have faith that it will help them. Also, I always kept my eyes on the prize that I'd defined for myself: to bring new and improved treatments to sick people. At the risk of immodesty, I defined my own values-based performance standards with others who shared these values, even as we operated in the ROI-driven (return on investment) realm of biopharma.

Contrary to the media's negative portrayal of drug makers, we sought to maintain our quest for excellence, uncompromising adherence to rigorous science, and an impeccable level of personal integrity in the business setting. We relied on solid judgement, broad medical knowledge, a high tolerance for risk, and a confident, optimistic belief that success was possible despite the odds. The results -- drugs that saved lives, conquered illness, and restored health. Not a bad day at the office!

CHAPTER 13
Reflections

Late in 1968, I was plucked out of my robust life and thrust into a world of disease, confusion, uncertainty, and fear. Before then, I was a high achiever with a promising future as a physician, working in a Montreal hospital as a medical resident. Though I was only twenty-four, being a doctor put me in a role of authority, with both patients and staff depending on my skills and ability to make important judgement calls and life-and-death decisions.

The flashing blue light I saw that November was not just a symptom; it was a hallmark of the stunning role reversal that was about to occur. For the next three months, I became a receiver of care, not a provider. I was vulnerable, needy, and sick and was dependent on the skills, ability, and judgement of others for any hope of getting my life back on track. The tables turned in an instant. One minute, I was an energetic hospital house officer, talking on the phone. The next minute, I awoke a hospital patient who had collapsed with a generalized seizure.

Thus began a three-month nightmare, spent mostly in two hospitals, including a psychiatric facility. Hard-working and straight as an arrow, I had never in my wildest dreams imagined myself as a psychiatric patient, much less a psychotic one who couldn't figure out which shoe to put on which foot. This terrifying ordeal was filled with personal torture, constant and sometimes agonizing tests, medications with mind-numbing side effects, and uncertainty of diagnosis and outcome. A calamitous illness threatened to shatter my health, along with my hopes, family plans, and professional aspirations.

For many patients, hospital time is an altered reality. That wasn't so much the case for me during my first hospital stay, even with the abrupt role reversal. I understood the medical procedures. I knew and trusted many of my providers, some of whom had been my med school professors at McGill University. I'm not trivializing the situation—I was wracked by fear that I had a fatal brain tumor. But my illness was unfolding in the framework of hospital medical care, a world that was second nature to me.

A sense of altered reality did set in, though, upon leaving the hospital. In my personal life and return to work, I was starting to misinterpret what was happening around me. Soon, anxiety, memory problems, and the beginnings of psychosis landed me back in the hospital. When the doctors saw my behavior growing increasingly bizarre, they transferred me to AMI, the psychiatric hospital where I remained for two months.

If I possess any memories of that miserable period on the psych ward, they're in a cellular vault in a deep, inaccessible corner of my brain. I only know it was miserable from research I conducted more than fifty years after the fact. With shock, I discovered how much suffering I endured—a result of symptoms, side effects, and the psychosis that unplugged my mind from reality. Hour by hour, day by day, I futilely struggled to piece together a cohesive picture from the fragmented, distorted, and delusional thoughts that had come uncontrolled in my mind. My heart grows heavy when I think of the worry and stress my illness created for my wife, parents, siblings, and friends.

LINGERING MYSTERIES

The 1950s and '60s saw big strides in the pharmaceutical treatment of mental illnesses. The groundbreaking drug chlorpromazine (brand names Largactil and Thorazine) was introduced into psychiatric practice due in part to the clinical research discoveries of Dr. Heinz E. Lehmann at McGill.[8] Chlorpromazine helped empty the psych wards of many thousands of psychotic patients who were able to go home safely, free of their debilitating symptoms. In 1957, Dr. Lehmann received the prestigious Albert Lasker Award for his seminal work with chlorpromazine and his contribution to psychiatry.[9]

By the time I became ill, doctors had grown quite liberal with the use of this new generation of drugs. At the peak of my illness, I was on at least six medicines, some with potent side effects, alone or in combination. I've wondered whether my two-month amnesia at AMI was the result of the illness, the heavy doses of medications, or both. Based on my review of current dosage recommendations, there's a good chance it was the meds.

Largactil, for instance, is now usually given at 50 to 100 mg. orally for severe psychosis. For weeks, I took 300 to 375 mg. of Largactil every day. I was also on Stelazine (trifluoperazine), which can have toxic effects, including memory loss, when taken alongside Largactil. My meds also caused the

---

[8.] Thomas A. Ban, "Fifty Years Chlorpromazine: A Historical Perspective," *Neuropsychiatric Disease and Treatment* 3, no. 4 (2007): 495, PMID: 19300578, PMCID: PMC2655089.

[9.] John M. Oldham, "Heinz. E. Lehmann, MD (1911–2000)," *Archives of General Psychiatry* 58, no. 12 (2001): 1178, https://doi.org/10.1001/archpsyc.58.12.1178.

noticeable side effects that mimic the symptoms of Parkinson's disease. But despite the negative side effects, it's likely these drugs contributed to my rapid improvement. Now I'm going to add something that seems contradictory. But please bear in mind that my condition was complex, the cause was uncertain, and doctors didn't have the advantages of today's technology with its superior tools for pinpointing the causes of brain disorders.

After a week or two at AMI, doctors increased my Largactil dose in advance of adding an antidepressant to my meds. Dr. Robert Allen Cleghorn, chair of the McGill psychiatry department, was a leading figure in North American psychiatry who had researched and published profusely.[10] Dr. Cleghorn visited me at AMI and, for reasons that are not apparent to me from my medical records, suggested that my medications be reduced. His advice was heeded. Not too long afterwards, I entered what I consider my recovery phase, which started gradually and picked up speed at a remarkable rate. There's no way to know what was responsible for this. Did the drugs control the psychosis and have a healing effect on my disordered brain? Was it the reduction in meds and their side effects that accelerated things? Or did I have a disease that just ran its natural course? It's another issue in the realm of the probable, not the proven.

I believe other factors also contributed to my miraculous recovery. First is the superb quality of care I received; MNH was a center of excellence for issues such as seizures, and AMI was a mecca for the use of psychopharmacology in McGill-affiliated hospitals. Second is the incredible support of Gloria, my family, and my friends. Third is my own

---

[10] D. J. Lewis and Frederick H. Lowy, "Robert A. Cleghorn, M.D.: The Well-Tempered Psychiatrist," *The Canadian Psychiatric Association Journal* 15, no. 6 (1970): 513, https://doi.org/10.1177/0706743770015006.

courage and tenacity; my sense of identity was linked to being a physician scientist, and I was determined to get back on the path to achieving my career goals and to my dream of having a wonderful family life with Gloria and our future children. The fourth factor was simply luck.

So what caused my illness in the first place? I'd like to wrap this up for you in a nice package tied up with ribbon and a pretty bow—a clear, definitive diagnosis to explain what launched this sudden cascade of harrowing events. Honestly, as a scientist, I'd appreciate such an indisputable answer myself. But scientists can't draw reliable conclusions from inconclusive data, and the evidence in this case doesn't support 100 percent certainty. The final diagnosis in my AMI discharge report was nonspecific: *acute brain syndrome—etiology unknown.*

There were several credible theories along the way. Fortunately, a brain tumor was ruled out fairly early in the process. The one theory that kept emerging consistently was that an organic disease caused my seizures and then my extreme psychiatric symptoms. The prime suspect was viral encephalitis. —brain inflammation resulting from a viral infection. There really isn't another tenable explanation for inflammation in the brain that gets better on its own. I think all of my doctors ultimately believed I had viral encephalitis.

More evidence lies in the fact that after my release, I never saw another flashing blue light, never had another seizure, and never had any more psychiatric symptoms. In today's world, this kind of viral infection can often be readily identified. Back then, we could only assume, not prove. I believe with a high degree of confidence that I had viral encephalitis, But no iron-clad guarantee.

TAKEAWAYS AND HIDDEN LESSONS

With time on my hands during the COVID-19 pandemic, I launched this project to satisfy my curiosity about a mystery illness that struck me in my twenties. The project transformed itself from a pure medical investigation into a journey of exploration. My research involved gathering written evidence of my illness and researching relevant medical information and contemporary standards of care from the late 1960s. Then I interviewed people close to me at the time, seeking any recollections they might have.

Besides investigating the medical details, I looked at how a health crisis that nearly destroyed my life may have continued to influence me after my stunning and complete recovery in 1969. I've stressed that education and lifelong learning are core values for Gloria and me. What I didn't expect was that writing this book would turn into more of an education for me rather than a simple reporting of events. Outside of the memory loss during my illness, I guess I assumed I was the foremost authority on Dr. Irving Fox. (OK, I may have to concede that title to Gloria!) But this process has proven to be a surprising learning experience as I reflected on the personal and professional choices I made and realized, retrospectively, how they were shaped by my illness.

Let's take a look at some of the lessons from my illness that may be of help to you or your loved ones in dealing with sickness or injury.

What happened to me can happen to anyone, regardless of age, state of health, or socioeconomic status. Denial may make you feel safe for the moment, but it's likely to do more harm than good. Try to accept the reality that change and uncertainty are unavoidable parts of life. That doesn't mean you're resigning yourself to fate. But if you spend your energy denying and resisting the truth, you won't have a clear head to process information and make sound decisions.

No matter how strong and vital you feel at the moment, life is more fragile than it seems. Circumstances can change instantly. The healthier you are when something goes wrong, the more resources you'll have to draw on for your recovery. So take good care of your body in terms of lifestyle—good diet, health screenings, exercise, vaccinations, safety precautions—you know the drill.

At the same time, make an effort to recognize each day, each choice you make, each interaction with a loved one, and every little contribution you make to the world as the precious gifts they are. Counting your blessings may sound like a cliché, but people who are thankful and optimistic tend to have better health outcomes than those who are angry, cynical, or aggrieved.

When a crisis hits, try not to assume the worst, as I did when I was sure I had a deadly brain tumor. One should always prepare for bad scenarios, but there's no mileage in catastrophizing. Keep an open mind about your diagnosis and treatment and, if you can, wait for the facts to come in before making critical decisions. Trust but verify. It's OK to request more information and ask your doctors to explain how they came to the conclusions they did about your care. Learn the side effects of any treatments, but don't necessarily make that the basis for refusing. Consider the risk/benefit ratio and whether the benefits of treating your disease or alleviating symptoms are greater than the risks of side effects.

Following my recovery, Gloria and I went on with our lives as if I'd never been sick. With the fast-moving pace of our lives, careers, and growing family, I put my illness in the past and forgot about it. In terms of my daily life, that's absolutely true. But in another sense, I could never erase the experience. Memories don't evaporate; they are information that's changed into a different format and stored in an out-of-the-way place, sort of like archiving an old email. I suspect that the memories of the trauma were imprinted in my brain and influenced my life in ways that I never contemplated before writing this book.

I believe that in my roles as physician, researcher, professor, husband, father, and engaged community member, I have been more compassionate, kind, respectful, patient, and determined as a result of my illness. I act with greater integrity, in ways that are more aligned with my values and principles. I think I was better able to clarify my values and goals, . Plus more comfortable with risk, and more tolerant of change and uncertainty.

I've described the moves we made as I switched jobs and careers, always with some level of risk and major changes requiring us to adapt. On two occasions, my job changes meant moving countries while Gloria was pregnant. Happily, Gloria is a high achiever who is smart, competent, well-organized, and a fabulous family manager. As much as I was passionately devoted to my work, my family is of equal, if not greater, importance to me. With her wisdom, intellectual capacity, support for me, and superb parenting skills, Gloria has been an incomparable life partner. She, too, suffered from my traumatic illness, yet her strength and vision helped steer us out of adversity, through recovery, and into a happy, fulfilling family life.

When I joined Biogen, I encountered a radically different type of business model; an intense new work culture; a difficult, demanding boss; and a revolving door of senior management personnel. After the financial risk of my first two years had passed, I could easily have found other work. Why did I remain when so many others had fled? Perhaps certain hidden lessons of my illness were embedded in my bones. I stayed because I'd identified my heart's-desire goal of developing new drugs to alleviate human suffering. I was loath to give up the accomplishments of the clinical work we were doing on Avonex with approval potential that might fulfill my goal. My illness had given me the emotional strength and endurance to tolerate uncertainties. My goals were more important to me than some discomfort in the workplace.

A three-month mystery illness that terrorized my family and me and literally drove me out of my mind ended up enriching my life more than I ever realized. Does that mean I'm grateful for the medical ordeal of a lifetime? No friggin' way! Unquestionably, I'd trade the whole wretched experience for a nice, uneventful afternoon in a Montreal movie theatre, humming along with the great Beatles tunes in *Yellow Submarine*. I wish I'd never gotten ill. But I did, and I accept that.

I am deeply grateful for a full recovery, the quality of care I received, the support and love of family and friends who helped me through, and for all the mentors and teachers who taught me so much. I'm grateful for the known and unknown ways my illness ultimately made me a stronger man and a better person—someone who could contribute to my community and society and, in a humble way, make the world a slightly better place. Perhaps this is my way of "paying it forward" and giving to others after the good fortune of getting my life back.

My calamitous illness is in the past. There is no flashing blue light! I was fortunate to recover and not miss a beat in my life. Now in my twilight years, I am satisfied that my gift of a lifetime was beneficial to me not only in my wonderful, productive, and loving family life but also beneficial to mankind through my professional career that brought unique medicines to treat terrible diseases. This story has a happy outcome and shows that it is possible to face horrible adversity and recover completely.

Works Cited

Antoine de Saint-Exupéry, The Little Prince, trans. Richard Howard (San Diego: Harcourt, 2000), 63.

D.J. Lewis and Frederick H. Lowy, "Robert A. Cleghorn, M.D.: The Well-Tempered Psychiatrist," The Canadian Psychiatric Association Journal 15, no. 6 (1970): 513, https://doi.org/10.1177/0706743770015006.

EW Holmes, Of rice and men: Bill Kelley's next generation. J Clin Invest 2005; 115, 2948-2952

Forrest Gump, directed by Robert Zemeckis (1994, Los Angeles, CA: Paramount Pictures, 2001), DVD.

J.D. Howell. The CT scan after 50 years-Continuity and change. New Eng. J Med 2021;385: 104-5.

John M. Oldham, "Heinz. E. Lehmann, MD (1911–2000)," Archives of General Psychiatry 58, no. 12 (2001): 1178, https://doi.org/10.1001/archpsyc.58.12.1178.

Michelle H. Silver, "The Good Fit—Why Medical Applicants' Personal Statements Are Anything but Personal," New England Journal of Medicine 384, no. 12 (March 25, 2021): 1086–1087, https://doi.org/10.1056/NEJMp2032383.

Robert Burns, "To a Mouse," in Poems, Chiefly in the Scottish Dialect (Kilmarnock: John Wilson, 1786), 138–140, https://digital.nls.uk/poems-chiefly-in-the-scottish-dialect/archive/74464614#?c.

Thomas A. Ban, "Fifty Years Chlorpromazine: A Historical Perspective," Neuropsychiatric Disease and Treatment 3, no. 4 (2007): 495, PMID: 19300578, PMCID: PMC2655089.

Thompson CN, Baumgartner J, Pichardo C, et al. COVID-19 Outbreak — New York City, February 29–June 1, 2020. MMWR Morbidity and Mortality Weekly Report 69 (November 20, 2020): 1725–1729, http://dx.doi.org/10.15585/mmwr.mm6946a2external icon.

Acknowledgments

This memoir encompasses a lifetime. A turning point was my calamitous illness from December 1968 to the end of February 1969, which is a key part of my story.

My beautiful soulmate, friend, and wife Gloria and I have been on a life journey together for more than fifty-six years, since we were married in June of 1966. During my illness she was my salvation and the purveyor of my hope. It's impossible to consider my life without her. I'm the dreamer, and she's the practical, independent stalwart who has kept me anchored to reality!

My parents, the late Nathan Fox and Phyllis Fox, were devoted parents who were involved with Gloria in managing many issues during my illness. Thank you to them for being pillars of support during my life.

My brother Allan was present throughout my illness and was caring and considerate while also finishing McGill med school and starting house officer training. He and my sister Rosanne Ain have been key presences and friends in my life. During my illness, Rosanne and her husband Steve were both in college and were "kids," as Rosanne said at the time.

My two precious friends Arnie Aberman and Lenny Diamond knew me before and during my illness, and we have continuing friendships to this day. They were both important to me during my illness. Arnie and I studied together and helped each other achieve a high level of excellence both in med school and during our house officer training. Lenny and I have known each other since the ninth grade, and he is now my cousin as well as being a wonderful lifetime friend!

I am grateful to my caregivers at the Montreal Neurological Hospital and the Allan Memorial Institute, McGill University teaching hospitals. My doctors and nurses were diligent in bringing me back to reality and recovering good health. Most of them have passed on, but they have left their indelible positive mark on me and my life. My nurses are the unsung heroes of my treatment and care, which is evident by their copious bedside notes, especially at AMI. These notes revealed to me my bizarre behaviors and suffering during my psychosis.

Doctors Francis McNaughton, Robert Cleghorn, and James Naiman were professors at McGill as well as incredible physicians who successfully cared for and treated me. They and many members of their teams were my teachers in medical school and famous for their scientific work.

Thank you to Michael Levin, my personal editor and writer. He made medical notes come alive through his narratives and the book come alive with contextual reality and empathy. I and my book benefitted from Michael's extraordinary skill and experience!

Jenn T. Grace and Bailly Morse guided me through finishing the book with standard formats, preparing it for publication and helping create strategies for effective distribution. I'm grateful for their support for me as a first-time author.

Book Club Questions

1. Why do you think that the author has chosen *The Flashing Light* as the title for this book?

2. Why is this book subtitled *A Medical Mystery Memoir*?

3. How did you react to Fox's response to *The Little Prince* book and the movie *Yellow Submarine*?

4. Given the bizarre behaviors of Fox during his psychosis, did you anticipate that he would recover completely?

5. Were you surprised by the numerous signs and symptoms caused by the antipsychotic medications that Fox took? What was your reaction to Dr. Cleghorn's recommendation to stop the medication?

6. It was unclear what made Fox get better: Did the disease run its course and improve on its own? Did the treatment with antipsychotic medication work? Was it due to Fox's strong family support, excellent doc-

tors, his determination, or a combination of all those factors? What do you believe made him better?

7. About his improvement, Fox says that he was grateful to 'get his life back'. Do you think that this influenced his career choices? Do you believe he consciously or subconsciously wanted to give back to mankind for this very positive outcome in his life?

8. How do you view Fox's switch from research in academic medicine to a career doing high-risk novel medicine development in the context of his recovery from a calamitous illness?

9. Do you think that Fox achieved his goal of giving back to others through the drug approvals accomplished by his project teams and his mentoring of colleagues?

10. Why do you think Irving and Gloria Fox did not reveal Fox's illness to people until after he retired? What does that say about society's view of mental illness in the 60s and 70s as compared to today?

11. How might people with their own calamitous personal events view Fox's severe illness and complete recovery?

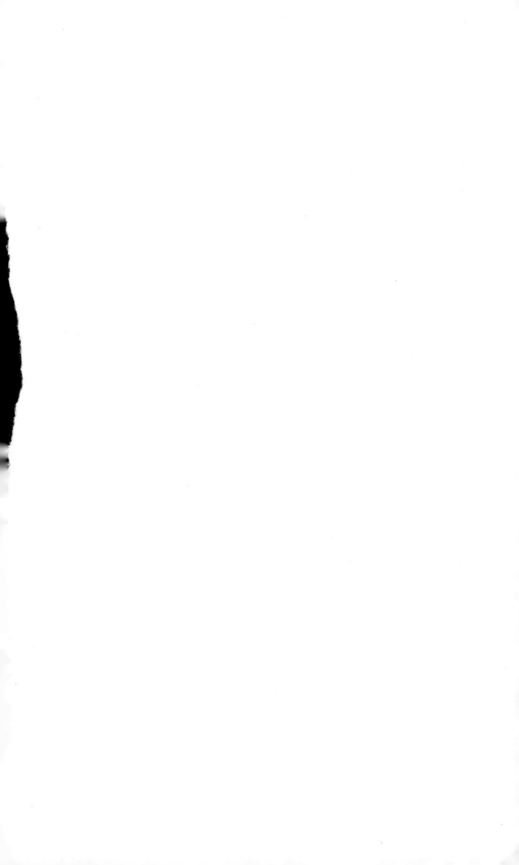

CPSIA information can be obtained
at www.ICGtesting.com
Printed in the USA
BVHW011251210423
662796BV00020B/885

9 798887 970073